BLACKWELL'S
UNDERGROUND CLINICAL VIGNETTES

MICROBIOLOGY
VOL. I, 3E

BLACKWELL'S
UNDERGROUND CLINICAL VIGNETTES

MICROBIOLOGY
VOL. I, 3E

VIKAS BHUSHAN, MD
University of California, San Francisco, Class of 1991
Series Editor, Diagnostic Radiologist

VISHAL PALL, MBBS
Government Medical College, Chandigarh, India, Class of 1996
Series Editor, U. of Texas, Galveston, Resident in Internal Medicine &
Preventive Medicine

TAO LE, MD
University of California, San Francisco, Class of 1996

HOANG NGUYEN, MD, MBA
Northwestern University, Class of 2001

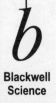

**Blackwell
Science**

CONTRIBUTORS

Sandra Mun
University of Texas Medical Branch, Class of 2002

Beth Ann Fair, MD
Eastern Virginia Medical School, Resident in Emergency Medicine

Kristen Lem Mygdal, MD
University of Kansas School of Medicine, Resident in Radiology

Mae Sheikh-Ali, MD
University of Damascus, Syria, Class of 1999

Shalin Patel, MD
McGraw Medical Center, Northwestern University, Resident in Internal Medicine

Jose M. Fierro, MD
La Salle University, Mexico City

FACULTY REVIEWER

Warren Levinson, MD, PHD
Professor of Microbiology and Immunology, UCSF School of Medicine

© 2002 by Blackwell Science, Inc.

Editorial Offices:
Commerce Place, 350 Main Street, Malden,
    Massachusetts 02148, USA
Osney Mead, Oxford OX2 0EL, England
25 John Street, London WC1N 2BS, England
23 Ainslie Place, Edinburgh EH3 6AJ, Scotland
54 University Street, Carlton, Victoria 3053,
    Australia

Other Editorial Offices:
Blackwell Wissenschafts-Verlag GmbH,
    Kurfürstendamm 57, 10707 Berlin, Germany
Blackwell Science KK, MG Kodenmacho Building,
    7-10 Kodenmacho Nihombashi, Chuo-ku,
    Tokyo 104, Japan
Iowa State University Press, A Blackwell Science
    Company, 2121 S. State Avenue, Ames, Iowa
    50014-8300, USA

Acquisitions: Laura DeYoung
Development: Amy Nuttbrock
Production: Lorna Hind and Shawn Girsberger
Manufacturing: Lisa Flanagan
Marketing Manager: Kathleen Mulcahy
Cover design by Leslie Haimes
Interior design by Shawn Girsberger
Typeset by TechBooks
Printed and bound by Capital City Press

Blackwell's Underground Clinical Vignettes:
    Microbiology I, 3e
ISBN 0-632-04547-7

Printed in the United States of America
02 03 04 05 5 4 3 2 1

First Indian Reprint 2002

Printed and bound by Multivista Global Limited,
Chennai - 600 042.

The Blackwell Science logo is a trade mark of
Blackwell Science Ltd., registered at the United
Kingdom Trade Marks Registry

Library of Congress Cataloging-in-Publication Data
Bhushan, Vikas.
Blackwell's underground clinical vignettes.
Microbiology / Author, Vikas Bhushan. – 3rd ed.
    p. ; cm. – (Underground clinical vignettes)
Rev. ed. of: Microbiology / Vikas Bhushan ... [et al.].
2nd ed. c1999-. ISBN 0-632-04547-7 (alk. paper)
1. Medical microbiology – Case studies.
2. Physicians – Licenses – United States –
Examinations – Study guides.
    [DNLM: 1. Microbiology – Case Report.
2. Microbiology – Problems and Exercises.
QW 18.2 B575b 2002] I. Title: Microbiology.
II. Title: Underground clinical vignettes.
Microbiology. III. Microbiology. IV. Title. V. Series.
    QR46 .B465 2002
    616'.01'076–dc21

                                            2001004932

Notice

The authors of this volume have taken care that the information contained herein is accurate and compatible with the standards generally accepted at the time of publication. Nevertheless, it is difficult to ensure that all the information given is entirely accurate for all circumstances. The publisher and authors do not guarantee the contents of this book and disclaim any liability, loss, or damage incurred as a consequence, directly or indirectly, of the use and application of any of the contents of this volume.

CONTENTS

ACKNOWLEDGMENTS

Throughout the production of this book, we have had the support of many friends and colleagues. Special thanks to our support team including Anu Gupta, Andrea Fellows, Anastasia Anderson, Srishti Gupta, Mona Pall, Jonathan Kirsch and Chirag Amin. For prior contributions we thank Gianni Le Nguyen, Tarun Mathur, Alex Grimm, Sonia Santos and Elizabeth Sanders.

We have enjoyed working with a world-class international publishing group at Blackwell Science, including Laura DeYoung, Amy Nuttbrock, Lisa Flanagan, Shawn Girsberger, Lorna Hind and Gordon Tibbitts. For help with securing images for the entire series we also thank Lee Martin, Kristopher Jones, Tina Panizzi and Peter Anderson at the University of Alabama, the Armed Forces Institute of Pathology, and many of our fellow Blackwell Science authors.

For submitting comments, corrections, editing, proofreading, and assistance across all of the vignette titles in all editions, we collectively thank:

Tara Adamovich, Carolyn Alexander, Kris Alden, Henry E. Aryan, Lynman Bacolor, Natalie Barteneva, Dean Bartholomew, Debashish Behera, Sumit Bhatia, Sanjay Bindra, Dave Brinton, Julianne Brown, Alexander Brownie, Tamara Callahan, David Canes, Bryan Casey, Aaron Caughey, Hebert Chen, Jonathan Cheng, Arnold Cheung, Arnold Chin, Simion Chiosea, Yoon Cho, Samuel Chung, Gretchen Conant, Vladimir Coric, Christopher Cosgrove, Ronald Cowan, Karekin R. Cunningham, A. Sean Dalley, Rama Dandamudi, Sunit Das, Ryan Armando Dave, John David, Emmanuel de la Cruz, Robert DeMello, Navneet Dhillon, Sharmila Dissanaike, David Donson, Adolf Etchegaray, Alea Eusebio, Priscilla A. Frase, David Frenz, Kristin Gaumer, Yohannes Gebreegziabher, Anil Gehi, Tony George, L.M. Gotanco, Parul Goyal, Alex Grimm, Rajeev Gupta, Ahmad Halim, Sue Hall, David Hasselbacher, Tamra Heimert, Michelle Higley, Dan Hoit, Eric Jackson, Tim Jackson, Sundar Jayaraman, Pei-Ni Jone, Aarchan Joshi, Rajni K. Jutla, Faiyaz Kapadi, Seth Karp, Aaron S. Kesselheim, Sana Khan, Andrew Pin-wei Ko, Francis Kong, Paul Konitzky, Warren S. Krackov, Benjamin H.S. Lau, Ann LaCasce, Connie Lee, Scott Lee, Guillermo Lehmann, Kevin Leung, Paul Levett, Warren Levinson, Eric Ley, Ken Lin,

Pavel Lobanov, J. Mark Maddox, Aram Mardian, Samir Mehta, Gil Melmed, Joe Messina, Robert Mosca, Michael Murphy, Vivek Nandkarni, Siva Naraynan, Carvell Nguyen, Linh Nguyen, Deanna Nobleza, Craig Nodurft, George Noumi, Darin T. Okuda, Adam L. Palance, Paul Pamphrus, Jinha Park, Sonny Patel, Ricardo Pietrobon, Riva L. Rahl, Aashita Randeria, Rachan Reddy, Beatriu Reig, Marilou Reyes, Jeremy Richmon, Tai Roe, Rick Roller, Rajiv Roy, Diego Ruiz, Anthony Russell, Sanjay Sahgal, Urmimala Sarkar, John Schilling, Isabell Schmitt, Daren Schuhmacher, Sonal Shah, Fadi Abu Shahin, Mae Sheikh-Ali, Edie Shen, Justin Smith, John Stulak, Lillian Su, Julie Sundaram, Rita Suri, Seth Sweetser, Antonio Talayero, Merita Tan, Mark Tanaka, Eric Taylor, Jess Thompson, Indi Trehan, Raymond Turner, Okafo Uchenna, Eric Uyguanco, Richa Varma, John Wages, Alan Wang, Eunice Wang, Andy Weiss, Amy Williams, Brian Yang, Hany Zaky, Ashraf Zaman and David Zipf.

For generously contributing images to the entire *Underground Clinical Vignette* Step 1 series, we collectively thank the staff at Blackwell Science in Oxford, Boston, and Berlin as well as:

- Axford, J. *Medicine.* Osney Mead: Blackwell Science Ltd, 1996. Figures 2.14, 2.15, 2.16, 2.27, 2.28, 2.31, 2.35, 2.36, 2.38, 2.43, 2.65a, 2.65b, 2.65c, 2.103b, 2.105b, 3.20b, 3.21, 8.27, 8.27b, 8.77b, 8.77c, 10.81b, 10.96a, 12.28a, 14.6, 14.16, 14.50.

- Bannister B, Begg N, Gillespie S. *Infectious Disease, 2nd Edition.* Osney Mead: Blackwell Science Ltd, 2000. Figures 2.8, 3.4, 5.28, 18.10, W5.32, W5.6.

- Berg D. *Advanced Clinical Skills and Physical Diagnosis.* Blackwell Science Ltd., 1999. Figures 7.10, 7.12, 7.13, 7.2, 7.3, 7.7, 7.8, 7.9, 8.1, 8.2, 8.4, 8.5, 9.2, 10.2, 11.3, 11.5, 12.6.

- Cuschieri A, Hennessy TPJ, Greenhalgh RM, Rowley DA, Grace PA. *Clinical Surgery.* Osney Mead: Blackwell Science Ltd, 1996. Figures 13.19, 18.22, 18.33.

- Gillespie SH, Bamford K. *Medical Microbiology and Infection at a Glance.* Osney Mead: Blackwell Science Ltd, 2000. Figures 20, 23.

- Ginsberg L. *Lecture Notes on Neurology, 7th Edition.* Osney Mead: Blackwell Science Ltd, 1999. Figures 12.3, 18.3, 18.3b.

- Elliott T, Hastings M, Desselberger U. *Lecture Notes on Medical Microbiology, 3rd Edition.* Osney Mead: Blackwell Science Ltd, 1997. Figures 2, 5, 7, 8, 9, 11, 12, 14, 15, 16, 17, 19, 20, 25, 26, 27, 29, 30, 34, 35, 52.

- Mehta AB, Hoffbrand AV. *Haematology at a Glance*. Osney Mead: Blackwell Science Ltd, 2000. Figures 22.1, 22.2, 22.3.

Please let us know if your name has been missed or misspelled and we will be happy to make the update in the next edition.

PREFACE TO THE 3RD EDITION

We were very pleased with the overwhelmingly positive student feedback for the 2nd edition of our *Underground Clinical Vignettes* series. Well over 100,000 copies of the UCV books are in print and have been used by students all over the world.

Over the last two years we have accumulated and incorporated **over a thousand "updates"** and improvements suggested by you, our readers, including:

- many additions of specific boards and wards testable content

- deletions of redundant and overlapping cases

- reordering and reorganization of all cases in both series

- a new master index by case name in each Atlas

- correction of a few factual errors

- diagnosis and treatment updates

- addition of 5–20 new cases in every book

- and the addition of clinical exam photographs within *UCV— Anatomy*

And most important of all, the third edition sets now include two brand new **COLOR ATLAS** supplements, one for each Clinical Vignette series.

- The *UCV–Basic Science Color Atlas* (*Step 1*) includes over 250 color plates, divided into gross pathology, microscopic pathology (histology), hematology, and microbiology (smears).

- The *UCV–Clinical Science Color Atlas* (*Step 2*) has over 125 color plates, including patient images, dermatology, and funduscopy.

Each atlas image is descriptively captioned and linked to its corresponding Step 1 case, Step 2 case, and/or Step 2 MiniCase.

How Atlas Links Work:

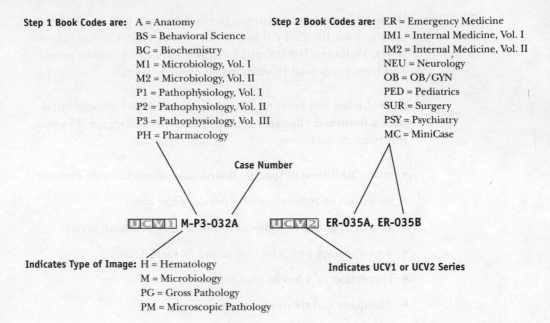

Step 1 Book Codes are:
- A = Anatomy
- BS = Behavioral Science
- BC = Biochemistry
- M1 = Microbiology, Vol. I
- M2 = Microbiology, Vol. II
- P1 = Pathophysiology, Vol. I
- P2 = Pathophysiology, Vol. II
- P3 = Pathophysiology, Vol. III
- PH = Pharmacology

Step 2 Book Codes are:
- ER = Emergency Medicine
- IM1 = Internal Medicine, Vol. I
- IM2 = Internal Medicine, Vol. II
- NEU = Neurology
- OB = OB/GYN
- PED = Pediatrics
- SUR = Surgery
- PSY = Psychiatry
- MC = MiniCase

Case Number

UCV1 M-P3-032A   UCV2 ER-035A, ER-035B

Indicates Type of Image:
- H = Hematology
- M = Microbiology
- PG = Gross Pathology
- PM = Microscopic Pathology

Indicates UCV1 or UCV2 Series

- If the Case number (032, 035, etc.) is not followed by a letter, then there is only one image. Otherwise A, B, C, D indicate up to 4 images.

Bold Faced Links: In order to give you access to the largest number of images possible, we have chosen to cross link the Step 1 and 2 series.

- If the link is bold-faced this indicates that the link is direct (i.e., Step 1 Case with the Basic Science Step 1 Atlas link).

- If the link is not bold-faced this indicates that the link is indirect (Step 1 case with Clinical Science Step 2 Atlas link or vice versa).

We have also implemented a few structural changes upon your request:

- Each current and future edition of our popular *First Aid for the USMLE Step 1* (Appleton & Lange/McGraw-Hill) and *First Aid for the USMLE Step 2* (Appleton & Lange/McGraw-Hill) book will be linked to the corresponding UCV case.

- We eliminated UCV → First Aid links as they frequently become out of date, as the *First Aid* books are revised yearly.

- The Color Atlas is also specially designed for quizzing—captions are descriptive and do not give away the case name directly.

We hope the updated UCV series will remain a unique and well-integrated study tool that provides compact clinical correlations to basic science information. They are designed to be easy and fun (comparatively) to read, and helpful for both licensing exams and the wards.

We invite your corrections and suggestions for the fourth edition of these books. For the first submission of each factual correction or new vignette that is selected for inclusion in the fourth edition, you will receive a personal acknowledgement in the revised book. If you submit over 20 high-quality corrections, additions or new vignettes we will also consider **inviting you to become a "Contributor" on the book of your choice**. If you are interested in becoming a potential "Contributor" or "Author" on a future UCV book, or working with our team in developing additional books, please also e-mail us your CV/resume.

We prefer that you submit corrections or suggestions via electronic mail to **UCVteam@yahoo.com**. Please include "Underground Vignettes" as the subject of your message. If you do not have access to e-mail, use the following mailing address: Blackwell Publishing, Attn: UCV Editors, 350 Main Street, Malden, MA 02148, USA.

Vikas Bhushan
Vishal Pall
Tao Le
October 2001

HOW TO USE THIS BOOK

This series was originally developed to address the increasing number of clinical vignette questions on medical examinations, including the USMLE Step 1 and Step 2. It is also designed to supplement and complement the popular *First Aid for the USMLE Step 1* (Appleton & Lange/McGraw Hill) and *First Aid for the USMLE Step 2* (Appleton & Lange/McGraw Hill).

Each UCV 1 book uses a series of approximately 100 **"supra-prototypical" cases as a way to condense testable facts and associations**. The clinical vignettes in this series are designed to incorporate as many testable facts as possible into a cohesive and memorable clinical picture. The vignettes represent composites drawn from general and specialty textbooks, reference books, thousands of USMLE style questions and the personal experience of the authors and reviewers.

Although each case tends to present all the signs, symptoms, and diagnostic findings for a particular illness, **patients generally will not present with such a "complete" picture either clinically or on a medical examination**. Cases are not meant to simulate a potential real patient or an exam vignette. All the **boldfaced "buzzwords" are for learning purposes** and are not necessarily expected to be found in any one patient with the disease.

Definitions of selected important terms are placed within the vignettes in (SMALL CAPS) in parentheses. Other parenthetical remarks often refer to the pathophysiology or mechanism of disease. The format should also help students learn to present cases succinctly during oral "bullet" presentations on clinical rotations. The cases are meant to serve as a condensed review, not as a primary reference. The information provided in this book has been prepared with a great deal of thought and careful research. This book should not, however, be considered as your sole source of information. Corrections, suggestions and submissions of new cases are encouraged and will be acknowledged and incorporated when appropriate in future editions.

ABBREVIATIONS

5-ASA	5-aminosalicylic acid
ABGs	arterial blood gases
ABVD	adriamycin/bleomycin/vincristine/dacarbazine
ACE	angiotensin-converting enzyme
ACTH	adrenocorticotropic hormone
ADH	antidiuretic hormone
AFP	alpha fetal protein
AI	aortic insufficiency
AIDS	acquired immunodeficiency syndrome
ALL	acute lymphocytic leukemia
ALT	alanine transaminase
AML	acute myelogenous leukemia
ANA	antinuclear antibody
ARDS	adult respiratory distress syndrome
ASD	atrial septal defect
ASO	anti-streptolysin O
AST	aspartate transaminase
AV	arteriovenous
BE	barium enema
BP	blood pressure
BUN	blood urea nitrogen
CAD	coronary artery disease
CALLA	common acute lymphoblastic leukemia antigen
CBC	complete blood count
CHF	congestive heart failure
CK	creatine kinase
CLL	chronic lymphocytic leukemia
CML	chronic myelogenous leukemia
CMV	cytomegalovirus
CNS	central nervous system
COPD	chronic obstructive pulmonary disease
CPK	creatine phosphokinase
CSF	cerebrospinal fluid
CT	computed tomography
CVA	cerebrovascular accident
CXR	chest x-ray
DIC	disseminated intravascular coagulation
DIP	distal interphalangeal
DKA	diabetic ketoacidosis
DM	diabetes mellitus
DTRs	deep tendon reflexes
DVT	deep venous thrombosis

EBV	Epstein–Barr virus
ECG	electrocardiography
Echo	echocardiography
EF	ejection fraction
EGD	esophagogastroduodenoscopy
EMG	electromyography
ERCP	endoscopic retrograde cholangiopancreatography
ESR	erythrocyte sedimentation rate
FEV	forced expiratory volume
FNA	fine needle aspiration
FTA-ABS	fluorescent treponemal antibody absorption
FVC	forced vital capacity
GFR	glomerular filtration rate
GH	growth hormone
GI	gastrointestinal
GM-CSF	granulocyte macrophage colony stimulating factor
GU	genitourinary
HAV	hepatitis A virus
hcG	human chorionic gonadotrophin
HEENT	head, eyes, ears, nose, and throat
HIV	human immunodeficiency virus
HLA	human leukocyte antigen
HPI	history of present illness
HR	heart rate
HRIG	human rabies immune globulin
HS	hereditary spherocytosis
ID/CC	identification and chief complaint
IDDM	insulin-dependent diabetes mellitus
Ig	immunoglobulin
IGF	insulin-like growth factor
IM	intramuscular
JVP	jugular venous pressure
KUB	kidneys/ureter/bladder
LDH	lactate dehydrogenase
LES	lower esophageal sphincter
LFTs	liver function tests
LP	lumbar puncture
LV	left ventricular
LVH	left ventricular hypertrophy
Lytes	electrolytes
MCHC	mean corpuscular hemoglobin concentration
MCV	mean corpuscular volume
MEN	multiple endocrine neoplasia

MGUS	monoclonal gammopathy of undetermined significance
MHC	major histocompatibility complex
MI	myocardial infarction
MOPP	mechlorethamine/vincristine (Oncovorin)/procarbazine/prednisone
MR	magnetic resonance (imaging)
NHL	non-Hodgkin's lymphoma
NIDDM	non-insulin-dependent diabetes mellitus
NPO	nil per os (nothing by mouth)
NSAID	nonsteroidal anti-inflammatory drug
PA	posteroanterior
PIP	proximal interphalangeal
PBS	peripheral blood smear
PE	physical exam
PFTs	pulmonary function tests
PMI	point of maximal intensity
PMN	polymorphonuclear leukocyte
PT	prothrombin time
PTCA	percutaneous transluminal angioplasty
PTH	parathyroid hormone
PTT	partial thromboplastin time
PUD	peptic ulcer disease
RBC	red blood cell
RPR	rapid plasma reagin
RR	respiratory rate
RS	Reed–Sternberg (cell)
RV	right ventricular
RVH	right ventricular hypertrophy
SBFT	small bowel follow-through
SIADH	syndrome of inappropriate secretion of ADH
SLE	systemic lupus erythematosus
STD	sexually transmitted disease
TFTs	thyroid function tests
tPA	tissue plasminogen activator
TSH	thyroid-stimulating hormone
TIBC	total iron-binding capacity
TIPS	transjugular intrahepatic portosystemic shunt
TPO	thyroid peroxidase
TSH	thyroid-stimulating hormone
TTP	thrombotic thrombocytopenic purpura
UA	urinalysis
UGI	upper GI
US	ultrasound

ID/CC	A 25-year-old **IV drug abuser** presents with a **high fever** with chills, malaise, a productive cough, hemoptysis, and right-sided pleuritic chest pain.
HPI	He also reports multiple skin infections at injection sites.
PE	VS: fever. PE: **stigmata of intravenous drug abuse** at multiple injection sites; skin infections; thrombosed peripheral veins; **splenomegaly and pulsatile hepatomegaly; ejection systolic murmur**, increasing with inspiration, heard in tricuspid area.
Labs	CBC: normochromic, normocytic anemia. UA: microscopic hematuria. Blood culture yields *Staphylococcus aureus*.
Imaging	Echo: presence of **vegetations on tricuspid valve** and **tricuspid incompetence**. CXR: consolidation.
Treatment	**High-dose intravenous penicillinase-resistant penicillin** in combination with an **aminoglycoside**. If the isolated *S. aureus* strain is **methicillin resistant, vancomycin** is the drug of choice.
Discussion	In drug addicts, the **tricuspid valve** is the site of infection more frequently (55%) than the aortic valve (35%) or the mitral valve (30%); these findings contrast markedly with the rarity of right-sided involvement in cases of infective endocarditis that are not associated with drug abuse. *Staphylococcus aureus* is responsible for the majority of cases. Certain organisms have a predilection for particular valves in cases of addict-associated endocarditis; for example, enterococci, other streptococcal species, and non-albicans *Candida* organisms predominantly affect the valves of the left side of the heart, while *S. aureus* infects valves on both the right and the left side of the heart. *Pseudomonas* organisms are associated with biventricular and multiple-valve infection in addicts. Complications of endocarditis include congestive heart failure, ruptured valve cusp, myocardial infarction, and myocardial abscess.
Atlas Link	U C V I PG-M1-001

1 **ACUTE BACTERIAL ENDOCARDITIS**

ID/CC A **25-year-old male** complains of increasing **shortness of breath** and **ankle edema** that have progressively worsened over the past 2 weeks.

HPI He also complains of fatigue, palpitations, and low-grade fever. His symptoms **followed a severe URI**. He denies any history of joint pain or skin rash (vs. rheumatic fever).

PE JVP elevated; pitting pedal edema; fine inspiratory crepitations heard at both lung bases; mild hepatosplenomegaly..

Labs ASO titers not elevated. CBC: lymphocytosis. ECG: first-degree AV block. ESR elevated; increased titers of antibodies to **coxsackievirus** demonstrated in serum.

Imaging CXR: **cardiomegaly** and **pulmonary edema**. Echo: **dilated cardiomyopathy with low ejection fraction**.

Gross Pathology Dilated heart with foci of epicardial, myocardial, and endocardial petechial hemorrhages.

Micro Pathology Endomyocardial biopsy reveals **diffuse infiltration by mononuclear cells**, predominantly lymphocytes; focal fibrosis.

Treatment Manage congestive heart failure and arrhythmias; cardiac transplant in intractable cases.

Discussion **Coxsackie B** is most often implicated in viral myocarditis. Nonviral causes of myocarditis include bacteria such as *Borrelia burgdorferi* (Lyme disease), parasites such as *Trypanosoma cruzi* (Chagas' disease), hypersensitivity reaction (systemic lupus erythematosus, drug reaction), radiation, and sarcoidosis; may also be idiopathic (giant cell myocarditis).

Atlas Link UCV1 M-M1-002

ID/CC A 35-year-old male complains of **fever, nonproductive cough**, and **chest pain**.

HPI He states that the chest pain developed after he had a severe cold for 1 week. He describes the pain as **severe, crushing, and constant** over the anterior chest and adds that it **worsens with inspiration** and is **relieved by sitting up** and bending forward.

PE VS: low-grade fever; sinus tachycardia. PE: triphasic **pericardial friction rub** (systolic and diastolic components followed by a third component in late diastole associated with atrial contraction); **elevated JVP**; inappropriate **increase in JVP with inspiration** (KUSSMAUL'S SIGN); pulsus paradoxus may also be seen.

Labs Moderately elevated transaminases and LDH; **elevated ESR; serum CPK-MB normal**. CBC: neutrophilic leukocytosis. ECG: **diffuse ST-segment elevation** (vs. myocardial infarction); **PR-segment depression**.

Imaging Echo: **pericardial effusion**. CXR: apparent **cardiomegaly** (due to effusion).

Gross Pathology In long-standing cases, pericardium may become fibrotic, scarred, and calcified.

Micro Pathology Pericardial biopsy reveals signs of acute inflammation with increased leukocytes, vascularity, and deposition of fibrin.

Treatment Analgesics for pain; steroids in resistant cases; indomethacin; surgical stripping of scarring in severe cases.

Discussion Acute pericarditis is commonly idiopathic. Known infectious causes include **coxsackievirus A and B, tuberculosis**, staphylococcal or pneumococcal infection, amebiasis, or actinomycosis; noninfectious causes include chronic renal failure, **collagen-vascular disease** (systemic lupus erythematosus, scleroderma, and rheumatoid arthritis), neoplasms, myocardial infarction, and trauma. Long-term sequelae include chronic constrictive pericarditis.

Atlas Link 🆄🅲🆅1 PG-M1-003

ID/CC A 64-year-old male presents with rapidly **progressive dyspnea and fever**.

HPI He has a history of orthopnea and paroxysmal nocturnal dyspnea and also reports pink, frothy sputum (HEMOPTYSIS). One month ago he underwent a **bioprosthetic valve replacement** for calcific aortic stenosis. He is not hypertensive and has never had overt cardiac failure in the past.

PE VS: fever; hypotension. PE: bilateral basal inspiratory crackles heard; cardiac auscultation suggestive of **aortic incompetence** (early diastolic murmur heard radiating down left sternal edge).

Labs CBC: normochromic, normocytic anemia. Three consecutive blood cultures yield **coagulase-negative *Staphylococcus epidermidis***; strain found to be **methicillin resistant**.

Imaging CXR (PA view): suggestive of **pulmonary edema**. Echo: confirms presence of **prosthetic aortic valve dehiscence** leading to incompetence and poor left ventricular function.

Treatment High-dose parenteral antibiotics—vancomycin (drug of choice for methicillin-resistant *S. aureus*), gentamicin, and oral rifampicin; surgical replacement of damaged prosthetic valve; prophylactic antibiotics (amoxicillin) for patients receiving oral/dental treatments to prevent transient bacteremia.

Discussion Prosthetic valve endocarditis is subdivided into two categories: early prosthetic valve endocarditis (EPVE), which becomes clinically manifest within 60 days after valve replacement (most commonly caused by *Staphylococcus epidermidis*, followed by gram-negative bacilli and *Candida*), and late prosthetic valve endocarditis (LPVE), which is manifested clinically more than 60 days after valve replacement (most commonly caused by viridans streptococci).

PROSTHETIC VALVE ENDOCARDITIS

ID/CC	A 25-year-old female complains of low-grade fever and myalgia of 3 weeks' duration.
HPI	She has a history of **rheumatic heart disease** (RHD). One month ago, she underwent a **dental extraction** and did not take the antibiotics that were prescribed for her.
PE	VS: fever. PE: pallor; small peripheral hemorrhages with slight nodular character (JANEWAY LESIONS); small, tender nodules on finger and toe pads (OSLER'S NODES); subungual linear streaks (SPLINTER HEMORRHAGES); petechial hemorrhages on conjunctiva, oral mucosa, and upper extremities; mild splenomegaly; apical diastolic murmur on cardiovascular exam; fundus exam shows oval retinal hemorrhages (ROTH'S SPOTS).
Labs	CBC/PBS: normocytic, normochromic anemia. UA: microscopic hematuria. Growth of penicillin-sensitive *Streptococcus viridans* on five of six blood cultures.
Imaging	Echo: vegetations along atrial surface of **mitral valve**.
Gross Pathology	Embolism from vegetative growths on valves may embolize peripherally (left-sided) or to the lung (right-sided).
Micro Pathology	Bacteria form nidus of infection in previously scarred or damaged valves; bacteria divide unimpeded once infection takes hold with further deposition of fibrin and platelets; peripheral symptoms such as Osler's nodes are believed to result from deposition of immune complexes.
Treatment	IV β-lactamase-resistant penicillin and gentamicin; bacteriostatic treatments ineffective.
Discussion	*S. viridans* is the most common cause of subacute infective endocarditis, while *Staphylococcus aureus* is the most common cause of acute bacterial endocarditis. Prophylactic antibiotics should be given to all RHD patients before any dental procedure. The disease continues to be associated with a high mortality rate.
Atlas Link	UCV1 PG-M1-005

SUBACUTE BACTERIAL ENDOCARDITIS

ID/CC	A 54-year-old female who **underwent** a left mastectomy with **axillary lymph node dissection** a year ago presents with **pain** together with rapidly spreading **redness** and **swelling** of the left **arm**.
HPI	One year ago, she was diagnosed and operated on for stage 1 **carcinoma of the left breast**.
PE	Left forearm swollen, indurated, pink, and markedly tender; overlying temperature raised; margins and borders of skin lesion ill defined and not elevated (vs. erysipelas).
Labs	Needle aspiration from advancing border of the lesion, when stained and cultured, isolated β-**hemolytic group A** streptococcus.
Treatment	Penicillinase-resistant penicillin (nafcillin/oxacillin).
Discussion	Cellulitis is an acute spreading infection of the skin that predominantly affects deeper subcutaneous tissue. **Group A streptococci and *Staphylococcus aureus*** are the **most common** etiologic agents in adults; *Haemophilus influenzae* infection is common in children. Patients with chronic venous stasis and lymphedema of any cause (lymphoma, filariasis, post–regional lymph node dissection, radiation therapy) are predisposed; recently, recurrent saphenous-vein donor-site cellulitis was found to be attributable to group A, C, or G streptococci.

ID/CC   A 16-year-old teenager presents to the outpatient clinic with a **painful facial rash** and **fever**.

HPI   One week ago, the patient went on a camping trip and scratched his face on some low-lying tree branches. There is no medical history of diabetes, cancer, or other chronic conditions.

PE   VS: **fever** (39.0°C); tachycardia (HR 110); BP normal. PE : **erythematous, warm, plaque-like rash** extending across cheeks and face bilaterally with **sharp, distinct borders** and **facial swelling**.

Labs   CBC: **leukocytosis** with **neutrophilia. ESR elevated**.

Treatment   **Antibiotics** with sufficient coverage for penicillinase-producing *Streptococcus* and *Staphylococcus* spp. (e.g., cephalexin); **analgesics/antipyretics**; elevate the affected part to reduce swelling.

Discussion   **Erysipelas** is an acute inflammation of the superficial layers of the connective tissues of the skin, usually on the face, almost always caused by infection with Group A *Streptococcus* which is part of normal bacterial skin flora. Risk factors include any breaks in the skin or **lymphedema**.

Atlas Link   󰁕󰁃󰂍󰀲 MC-136

7   **ERYSIPELAS**

ID/CC A 30-year-old **slaughterhouse worker** presents with a **painful red swelling** of the **index finger** of his right hand.

HPI The swelling developed 4 days after he was **injured** with a knife **while slaughtering a pig**.

PE Well-defined, exquisitely tender, slightly elevated **violaceous lesion seen on right index finger**; no suppuration noted; right epitrochlear and right axillary lymphadenopathy noted.

Labs Biopsy from edge of lesion yields *Erysipelothrix rhusiopathiae*, a thin, pleomorphic, nonsporulating, microaerophilic gram-positive rod.

Treatment **Penicillin G** or ciprofloxacin in penicillin-allergic patients.

Discussion Erysipeloid refers to **localized cellulitis**, usually of the fingers and hands, caused by *Erysipelothrix rhusiopathiae*; infection in humans is usually the result of **contact with infected animals** or their products (**often fish**). Organisms gain entry via cuts and abrasions on the skin.

ID/CC A **10-year-old** male complains of a spreading **skin rash** and **painful** swelling of both **wrists**.

HPI The patient's mother states that the rash began with **erythema of the cheeks** ("SLAPPED-CHEEK APPEARANCE") and subsequently progressed to involve the trunk and limbs.

PE **Erythematous lacy/reticular skin rash** involving face, trunk, and limbs; bilateral swelling and painful restriction of movement at both **wrist joints**.

Labs Serology detects presence of **specific IgM antibody to parvovirus**; ASO titer (to rule out acute rheumatic fever) normal; rheumatoid factor (to rule out rheumatoid arthritis) negative.

Treatment Self-limiting disease.

Discussion A small (20- to 26-nm), **single-stranded DNA virus, parvovirus B19** causes erythema infectiosum (fifth disease) in schoolchildren, **aplastic crises** in persons with underlying hemolytic disorders (e.g., sickle cell anemia), **chronic anemia** in immunocompromised hosts, arthralgia/arthritis in normal individuals, and **fetal loss** in pregnant women.

Atlas Link `UCV2` MC-299

ID/CC A **5-year-old** white male presents with golden-yellow, crusted lesions around his mouth and behind his ears.

HPI He has a history of intermittent low-grade fever, frequent "nose picking," and purulent discharge from his lesions. He has no history of hematuria (due to increased risk of poststreptococcal glomerulonephritis).

PE Characteristic **"honey-colored" crusted lesions** seen at **angle of mouth**, around nasal orifices, and behind ears.

Labs **Gram-positive cocci in chains** (STREPTOCOCCI) in addition to pus cells on Gram stain of discharge; β-hemolytic streptococci (group A streptococci) on blood agar culture; ASO titer negative.

Gross Pathology Erythematous lesions surrounding natural orifices with whitish or yellowish purulent exudate and crust formation.

Micro Pathology Inflammatory infiltrate of PMNs with varying degrees of necrosis.

Treatment Cephalosporin, penicillin, or erythromycin if allergic.

Discussion Impetigo is a highly communicable infectious disease that is most often caused by group A streptococci, occurs primarily in preschoolers, and may predispose to glomerulonephritis. It occurs most commonly on the face (periorbital area), hands, and arms. *Staphylococcus aureus* may coexist or cause bullous impetigo; group B streptococcal impetigo may be seen in newborns.

ID/CC A 30-year-old male homosexual visits his family doctor complaining of a nonpruritic **skin eruption** on his **upper limbs, trunk**, and **anogenital area**.

HPI He has been **HIV positive** for about 3 years and admits to having continued unprotected intercourse.

PE Multiple painless, pearly-white, dome-shaped, waxy, **umbilicated nodules** 2 to 5 mm in diameter on arms, trunk, and anogenital area; **palms and soles spared**.

Gross Pathology Firm, umbilicated nodules containing thick yellowish material.

Micro Pathology Stained histologic sections confirm diagnosis with large **cytoplasmic inclusions** (MOLLUSCUM BODIES) in material expressed from lesions.

Treatment Lesions may resolve spontaneously or be removed by curettage, cryotherapy, or podophyllin; no antiviral drug or vaccine available.

Discussion Molluscum contagiosum is a benign, autoinoculable skin disease of children and young adults; it is caused by a poxvirus (DNA virus) and is transmitted through sexual contact, close bodily contact, clothing, or towels. It is one of many opportunistic infections seen in AIDS patients (difficult to eradicate).

Atlas Link UCV2 MC-143

ID/CC	A 30-year-old black male presents with a nonpruritic **skin rash on the trunk, upper arm, and neck**.
HPI	The patient is otherwise in excellent health.
PE	Multiple **hypopigmented, scaling, confluent macules** seen on **trunk, upper arms, and neck**; no sensory loss demonstrated over areas of hypopigmentation; **Wood's lamp** examination of skin macules displays a **pale yellow to blue-white fluorescence**.
Labs	Examination of KOH mounting of scales from lesions demonstrates the presence of short, thick, tangled hyphae with clusters of large, spherical budding yeast cells with characteristic **"spaghetti-and-meatballs"** appearance.
Treatment	**Topical selenium sulfide**; antifungal agents such as **miconazole** and **clotrimazole**; oral itraconazole in recalcitrant cases.
Discussion	Pityriasis versicolor, which is common in young adults, is a relatively asymptomatic superficial skin infection caused by the lipophilic fungal organism *Pityrosporum orbiculare* (also termed *Malassezia furfur*). The lesions, which usually have a follicular origin, are small, hypopigmented-to-tan macules with a branlike scale; the macules are distributed predominantly on areas of the **upper trunk, neck**, and **shoulders**.
Atlas Links	UCV1 M-M1-012 UCV2 MC-148

ID/CC An **18-month-old** male is brought to the pediatrician following the appearance of an extensive skin rash.

HPI Four days ago he suddenly developed a **very high fever** (40°C) with no other symptoms or signs. The fever continued for 4 days until the day of his admission, when it abruptly **disappeared, coinciding with the onset of the rash**.

PE **Child looks well**; in no acute distress; **generalized rash** apparent as discrete 2- to 5-mm **rose-pink macules and papules on trunk, neck, and extremities** (face is spared); lesions blanch on pressure; no lymphadenopathy; splenomegaly may also be present.

Labs CBC/PBS: WBCs variable; relative lymphocytosis with atypical lymphocytes.

Treatment Supportive; foscarnet.

Discussion Roseola infantum, also called **exanthem subitum**, is caused by **human herpesvirus 6**. It is the most common exanthematous disease in infants 2 years of age or younger and is a frequent cause of **febrile convulsions**.

ID/CC	A **2-month-old** female infant presents with extensive **bullae** and large areas of denuded skin.
HPI	Her mother had suffered from **staphylococcal mastitis** 1 week ago.
PE	VS: fever. PE: large areas of red, painful, denuded skin on periorbital and peribuccal areas; flaccid bullae with **easy dislodgment of epidermis under pressure** (NIKOLSKY'S SIGN); mucosal surfaces largely uninvolved.
Labs	Vesicle fluid sterile; *Staphylococcus aureus* on blood culture.
Treatment	IV penicillinase-resistant penicillin (e.g., nafcillin, oxacillin). Treat with erythromycin if patient is allergic to penicillin.
Discussion	Scalded skin syndrome is caused by the exfoliating effect of **staphylococcal exotoxin**. The action of the exotoxin is to degrade desmoglein in desmosomes in the skin.

SCALDED SKIN SYNDROME

ID/CC	A 30-year-old man presents with a bilateral **red pruritic** skin **eruption** in the **groin** area.
PE	Bilateral, **circular papulosquamous skin eruption** on erythematous base with **active**, advancing **peripheral (serpiginous) border** over scrotum and perineum.
Labs	Microscopic examination reveals long septate **hyphae on KOH** skin scrapings.
Treatment	Topical antifungal agents (Whitfield's ointment, clotrimazole, miconazole); systemic therapy with oral griseofulvin, ketoconazole, or itraconazole in resistant cases.
Discussion	Tinea cruris and tinea corporis (COMMON RINGWORM) occur sporadically; *Trichophyton rubrum* is the most common cause. The inflammatory form, which is usually localized to the limbs, chest, or back, is commonly caused by *Microsporum canis* or *Trichophyton mentagrophytes*. Ringworm of the scalp, known as tinea capitis, is commonly seen in children and is caused by *Trichophyton tonsurans*.
Atlas Link	UCV2 MC-151

TINEA CORPORIS (RINGWORM)

ID/CC A 28-year-old male presents with a **red, pruritic skin eruption** on his trunk and his upper and lower limbs of a few hours' duration.

HPI One day earlier, he was prescribed cotrimoxazole for a UTI. He has not experienced any dyspnea.

PE Erythematous, warm, urticarial wheals (hives) seen over trunk, legs, and arms; no angioedema or respiratory distress.

Labs CBC: leukocytosis with eosinophilia. No parasites revealed on stool exam.

Gross Pathology Linear or oval, **raised papules or plaque-like wheals** up to several centimeters in diameter.

Micro Pathology Wide separation of dermal collagen fibers with dilatation of lymphatics and venules.

Treatment Topical agents to reduce itching; avoidance of causative agent (in this case, cotrimoxazole); antihistamines (primarily H_1 blockers but also H_2 blockers); consider glucocorticoids.

Discussion Mast cells and basophils are focal to urticarial reaction. When stimulated by certain immunologic or nonimmunologic mechanisms, storage granules in these cells release histamine and other mediators, such as kinins and leukotrienes. These agents produce the localized vasodilatation and transudation of fluid that characterize urticaria.

Atlas Link UCV2 MC-021

ID/CC A 7-year-old male is brought to his family physician complaining of a **thick yellowish discharge in his eyes that prevents him from opening his eyes in the morning**; for the past few days, his eyes have been **blood-red, painful**, and **watery**. His eye pain is exacerbated by exposure to light (PHOTOPHOBIA).

HPI Three of his classmates and a neighbor had a similar episode about 7 days ago (suggesting a **local epidemic** of such cases).

PE VS: no fever. PE: **normal visual acuity; erythematous palpebral conjunctiva**; watery eyes; **remains of thick mucus** found on inner canthal area; no corneal infiltrate on slit-lamp exam; normal anterior chamber; **mild preauricular lymphadenopathy**.

Labs Stained conjunctival smears reveal **lymphocytes**, giant cells, **neutrophils**, and bacteria.

Treatment Topical antimicrobial eye drops; cool compresses; minimize contact with others to avoid spread; avoid use of topical steroid preparations, as these can exacerbate bacterial and viral eye infections.

Discussion Conjunctivitis is a common disease of childhood that is mostly viral **(adenovirus)** and self-limiting; it occurs in epidemics, and secondary bacterial infections (staphylococci and streptococci) may result. Visual acuity is not affected.

17 **ACUTE CONJUNCTIVITIS**

ID/CC	A 35-year-old woman complains of fever and **pain in the face and upper teeth** (maxillary sinus), especially while leaning forward.
HPI	She has had a chronic cough, **nasal congestion, and discharge** for the past few months.
PE	VS: fever. PE: halitosis; greenish-yellow **postnasal discharge**; bilateral **boggy nasal mucosa**; bilateral percussion tenderness and **erythema over zygomatic arch; clouding of sinuses by transillumination**; dental and cranial nerve exams normal.
Labs	Nasal cultures reveal *Streptococcus pneumoniae*.
Imaging	CT, sinus: partial opacification of maxillary sinus with air-fluid level.
Gross Pathology	Erythematous and edematous nasal mucosa.
Micro Pathology	Presence of organisms and leukocytes in mucosa.
Treatment	Oral decongestants; amoxicillin, Bactrim, or fluoroquinolone.
Discussion	Other pathogens include other streptococci, *Haemophilus influenzae*, and *Moraxella*. The obstruction of ostia in the anterior ethmoid and middle meatal complex by retained secretions, mucosal edema, or polyps promotes sinusitis. *Staphylococcus aureus* and gram-negative species may cause chronic sinusitis. Fungal sinusitis may mimic chronic bacterial sinusitis. Complications include orbital cellulitis and abscesses.

ACUTE SINUSITIS

ID/CC	A 17-year-old boy presents with **itchy eyes**, nasal stuffiness, increased lacrimation, **sneezing**, and a **watery nasal discharge**.
HPI	He has had similar episodes in the past that have corresponded with **changing of the seasons**. His mother is known to have bronchial asthma.
PE	VS: no fever. PE: pallor; **boggy nasal mucosa; nasal polyps present**; conjunctiva congested; no exudate.
Labs	Conjunctival and nasal smear demonstrates presence of **eosinophils**; no bacteria on Gram stain; no neutrophils. Allergen skin tests (sensitized cutaneous mast cells) show positive sensitivity.
Gross Pathology	Nasal mucosa hyperemic and swollen with fluid transudation.
Micro Pathology	Local tissue inflammation and dysfunction of upper airway because of type I, IgE-mediated hypersensitivity response.
Treatment	Oral decongestants with intranasal corticosteroids; antihistamines; intranasal cromolyn sodium, especially before anticipated contact with allergen.
Discussion	Allergic rhinitis is commonly caused by exposure to **pollens**, dust content, and insect matter; symptoms are mediated by the release of vasoactive and chemotactic mediators from mast cells and basophils (e.g., histamine and leukotrienes) with IgE surface receptors.

ALLERGIC RHINITIS (HAY FEVER)

ID/CC	A 20-year-old male presents with a **runny nose, nasal congestion, sore throat, headache, and sneezing**.
HPI	He notes that his wife currently has similar symptoms.
PE	VS: mild fever. PE: rhinorrhea; congested and inflamed posterior pharyngeal wall; no lymphadenopathy.
Labs	Routine tests normal; routine throat swab staining and culture negative for bacteria.
Gross Pathology	Nasal membranes **edematous and erythematous** with watery discharge.
Micro Pathology	Mononuclear inflammation of mucosa; focal desquamation.
Treatment	Symptomatic.
Discussion	Colds occur 2 to 3 times a year in the average person in the United States; the peak incidence is in the winter months. **Rhinoviruses** account for the majority of viral URIs, followed by coronaviruses. Spread occurs by **direct contact** and respiratory droplets.

COMMON COLD (VIRAL RESPIRATORY INFECTION)

ID/CC A 60-year-old male presents with **swelling and a vesicular skin eruption on the left side of his face**.

HPI The patient reports that before the rash developed, he had severe radiating pain on the left side of his face. He also recalls having suffered an attack of **chickenpox during his childhood**.

PE **Unilateral vesicular rash** over left forehead and nasal bridge, including the tip of the nose, indicating involvement of the **nasociliary branch** of the trigeminal nerve (HUTCHINSON'S SIGN); skin of lids red and edematous; slit-lamp examination reveals numerous rounded spots composed of minute white dots involving epithelium and stroma, producing a **coarse subepithelial punctate keratitis; cornea** is **insensitive**.

Micro Pathology Vesicular skin lesions with **herpesvirus inclusions** that are **intranuclear and acidophilic** with a clear halo around them (**Cowdry type A inclusion bodies**); syncytial giant cells also seen.

Treatment **Acyclovir; steroids; cycloplegics**. Trifluorothymidine for HSV keratitis.

Discussion Herpes zoster ophthalmicus is caused by the **varicella zoster virus**, which causes chickenpox as a primary infection. Zoster is believed to be a **reactivation of the latent viral infection**. In **zoster ophthalmicus**, the chief **focus of reactivation is the trigeminal ganglion**, from which the virus travels down one or more branches of the ophthalmic division such that its area of distribution is marked out by rows of vesicles or scars left by the vesicles. **Ocular complications** arise during subsidence of the rash and are generally **associated with** involvement of the **nasociliary branch** of the trigeminal nerve.

ID/CC   An 18-year-old male complains of severe **irritation** in the left eye, **blurred vision**, excessive **lacrimation, and photophobia**.

HPI   He reports that he has had **similar episodes** in the past that were treated with an antiviral drug. His records indicate that he suffered the **first attack** at the age of 7, at which time his condition was diagnosed and treated **as a severe follicular keratoconjunctivitis**; his records also indicate a history of **recurrent** episodes of **herpes labialis**.

PE   Examination of left eye reveals circumcorneal congestion; fluorescein staining of cornea reveals infiltrates spreading in all directions, coalescing with each other and forming a **large, shallow ulcer with crenated edges** ("DENDRITIC ULCER"); **cornea** is **insensitive**.

Labs   HSV-1 demonstrated on immunofluorescent staining of epithelial scrapings as well as in the aqueous humor.

Treatment   **Trifluridine eye drops**; acyclovir has been shown to decrease recurrences.

Discussion   Most ocular herpetic infections are **caused by HSV-1**. It is also the primary cause of corneal blindness in the United States. Primary infections present as unilateral follicular conjunctivitis, blepharitis, or corneal epithelial opacities; **recurrences** may take the **form of keratitis** (> 90% of cases are unilateral), blepharitis, or keratoconjunctivitis. **Branching dendritic ulcers**, usually detected by fluorescein staining, are virtually diagnostic; deep stromal involvement may result in scarring, corneal thinning, and abnormal vascularization with resulting blindness or rupture of the globe.

ID/CC	A 20-year-old male swimmer complains of severe **pain** and **itching** in the right ear that is associated with a slight amount of **yellowish** (PURULENT) **discharge**.
HPI	The patient has no previous history of discharge from the ear and no history of associated deafness or tinnitus.
PE	Red, swollen area seen in right external auditory meatus that is partially obliterating the lumen; **movement of tragus** is exquisitely **painful** (TRAGAL SIGN).
Labs	Gram stain of aural swab reveals presence of gram-negative rods; culture isolates *Pseudomonas aeruginosa.*
Gross Pathology	Red, swollen area seen in cartilaginous part of external auditory meatus; when visualized, tympanic membrane is erythematous and moves normally with pneumatic otoscopy (vs. acute otitis media).
Treatment	**Eardrops** (either a combination of polymyxin, neomycin, and hydrocortisone or ofloxacin); gentle removal of debris in ear.
Discussion	Otitis externa is most common in summer months and is thought to arise from a change in the milieu of the external auditory meatus by increased alkalization and excessive moisture; this leads to bacterial overgrowth, most commonly with gram-negative rods such as *Pseudomonas* (also causes malignant otitis externa) and *Proteus* or fungi such as *Aspergillus.*

ENT/OPHTHALMOLOGY

ID/CC	An 18-month-old white female presents with **irritability** together with a bilateral, profuse, and foul-smelling **ear discharge** of 2 months' duration.
HPI	The patient had **recurrent URIs** last year, but her mother did not administer the complete course of antibiotics. The patient's mother has a history of feeding her child while lying down.
PE	Bilateral greenish-white ear discharge; **perforated tympanic membranes** in anteroinferior quadrant of both ears; **diminished mobility of tympanic membrane** on pneumatic otoscopy.
Labs	Gram-negative coccobacilli on Gram stain of discharge from tympanocentesis; *Haemophilus influenzae* seen on culture.
Gross Pathology	Possible complications include **ingrowth of squamous epithelium on upper middle ear** (CHOLESTEATOMA) if long-standing; conductive hearing loss; mastoiditis; and brain abscess.
Micro Pathology	Hyperemia and edema of inner ear and throat mucosa; hyperemia of tympanic membrane; deposition of cholesterol crystals in keratinized epidermoid cells in cholesteatoma.
Treatment	Keep ear dry; **amoxicillin-clavulanic acid**; surgical drainage for severe otalgia; myringoplasty.
Discussion	Otitis media is the most common pediatric bacterial infection and is caused by *Escherichia coli, Staphylococcus aureus*, and *Klebsiella pneumoniae* in neonates; in older children it is usually caused by pneumococcus (*Streptococcus pneumoniae*), *H. influenzae, Moraxella catarrhalis*, and group A streptococcus. Resistant strains are becoming increasingly common.

ID/CC	A 6-year-old male presents with complaints of a **mild sore throat and eye irritation**.
HPI	His mother says that he has spent hours at the **community swimming pool** this summer.
PE	Mild **rhinopharyngitis**; bilateral **conjunctival congestion** with scanty mucoid discharge.
Labs	Viral culture of conjunctival and nasopharyngeal swab yields **adenovirus**.
Treatment	No specific treatment; self-limiting illness.
Discussion	Adenovirus infections occur most often in **infants and young children**, who acquire the virus by the **respiratory or fecal-oral** route. The most common respiratory tract syndrome in this age group is mild coryza with pharyngitis; in older children, these symptoms may be accompanied by conjunctivitis. May also cause hemorrhagic cystitis in children. On electron microscopy it is seen as a **double-stranded nonenveloped DNA virus** surrounded by a 20-faced icosahedral protein capsid from which 12 antenna-like fibers or pentons extend radially.

ID/CC A 9-year-old male complains of **pain during swallowing** (ODYNOPHAGIA) for 2 days, accompanied by muscle aches, headache, and fever.

HPI He has otherwise been in good health.

PE VS: fever. PE: moderate erythema of pharynx; enlarged, **erythematous tonsils** covered with white **exudate**; tender cervical adenopathy.

Labs CBC: neutrophilic leukocytosis. ***Streptococcus pyogenes*** isolated on throat swab and culture.

Gross Pathology Hyperemia and swelling of upper respiratory tract mucosa; cryptic enlargement of tonsils with purulent exudate; enlargement of regional lymph nodes.

Micro Pathology Acute inflammatory response with polymorphonuclear infiltrate, hyperemia and edema with pus formation; hyperplasia of regional lymph nodes; dilatation of sinusoids.

Treatment **Oral penicillin V.**

Discussion Streptococcal pharyngitis is an acute bacterial infection produced by gram-positive **cocci in chains** (*Streptococcus*); pharyngitis is most commonly caused by group A streptococcus. Complications due to immune-mediated cross-reactivity and molecular mimicking may include glomerulonephritis and rheumatic fever.

Atlas Link 〔UCVI〕 M-M1-026

ID/CC	A **30-year-old female** presents to the surgical ER complaining of a stabbing **right upper quadrant abdominal pain**.
HPI	She is a prostitute who has been receiving treatment for **gonococcal pelvic inflammatory disease**.
PE	Right upper quadrant tenderness; cervical motion tenderness and mucopurulent cervicitis found on pelvic exam.
Labs	Cervical swab staining and culture identifies *Neisseria gonorrhoeae*.
Imaging	US: no evidence of cholecystitis. Peritoneoscopy: presence of **"violin string" adhesions between liver capsule and peritoneum**.
Gross Pathology	Adhesions noted between liver capsule and peritoneum.
Treatment	Antibiotic therapy (ceftriaxone and doxycycline) for patient (and for partner if warranted).
Discussion	**Acute fibrinous perihepatitis** (FITZ–HUGH–CURTIS SYNDROME) occurs as a complication of **gonococcal and chlamydial pelvic inflammatory disease** and clinically mimics cholecystitis.

GASTROENTEROLOGY

ID/CC	A 25-year-old male presents with sudden-onset, severe **vomiting**, nausea, **abdominal cramps, and diarrhea**.
HPI	He had returned home about 2 hours after attending a birthday party at which **meat and milk** were served in various forms. The **friend** who was celebrating his birthday **reported similar symptoms**.
PE	VS: **no fever**. PE: mild dehydration; diffuse abdominal tenderness; increased bowel sounds.
Labs	**Toxigenic staphylococcus** recovered from culturing food. Coagulase-positive staphylococcus cultured from **nose of one of the cooks** at party.
Micro Pathology	No mucosal lesions.
Treatment	Fluid and electrolyte balance; antibiotics not indicated.
Discussion	*Staphylococcus aureus* food poisoning results from the ingestion of food containing **preformed heat-stable enterotoxin B**. Outbreaks of staphylococcal food poisoning occur when **food handlers** who have contaminated superficial wounds or who are shedding infected nasal droplets inoculate foods such as meat, dairy products, salad dressings, cream sauces, and custard-filled pastries. The **incubation period** ranges from **2 to 8 hours**; the disease is self-limited.

ID/CC	An 11-year-old white male presents with **jaundice** and **dark yellow urine** that has been present for the last several days.
HPI	He also complains of nausea, vomiting, and malaise. For the past 2 weeks, he has had a low-grade fever and mild abdominal pain. He recently returned from a **vacation in Mexico**, where he said he consumed a lot of **shellfish**.
PE	Icterus; tender, firm hepatomegaly; no evidence of splenomegaly or free fluid in the peritoneal cavity.
Labs	**Direct hyperbilirubinemia**; elevated serum transaminases (ALT > AST); moderately elevated alkaline phosphatase; prolonged PT; increased urinary urobilinogen and bilirubin; **positive IgM antibody to hepatitis A (HAV)** indicative of active HAV infection.
Gross Pathology	May often appear normal.
Micro Pathology	Multifocal hepatocellular necrosis with Councilman bodies; lymphocytic infiltrates around necrotic foci; loss of lobular architecture.
Treatment	Supportive management; passive vaccination available.
Discussion	In hepatitis A infection, virus is shed 14 to 21 days before the onset of **jaundice**; patients are no longer infectious 7 days after the onset of jaundice. It is spread by **fecal-oral transmission** and is endemic in areas where there are **contaminated water sources**. There is **no chronic carrier state**; recovery takes place in 6 to 12 months. HAV is a naked, single-stranded RNA virus of the **picorna** family. A killed vaccine is available; passive immunization in the form of immune serum globulins is also available.

ID/CC	A 25-year-old male medical student presents with **jaundice** and **dark yellow urine**.
HPI	He admits to having experienced an accidental **needle stick** 2 months ago, which he did not report. He also complains of nausea, low-grade fever, and loss of appetite.
PE	Icterus; tender, firm **hepatomegaly**; no evidence of ascites or splenomegaly.
Labs	**Direct hyperbilirubinemia**; elevated serum transaminases (ALT > AST); mildly elevated alkaline phosphatase; **HBsAg positive; IgM anti-HBc positive** (present during window period).
Imaging	US, abdomen: hepatomegaly; increased echogenicity.
Gross Pathology	Liver may be enlarged, congested, or jaundiced; in fulminant cases of massive hepatic necrosis, liver becomes small, shrunken, and soft (acute yellow atrophy).
Micro Pathology	Liver biopsy reveals hepatocellular necrosis with **Councilman bodies** and ballooning degeneration; inflammation of portal areas with infiltration of mononuclear cells (small lymphocytes, plasma cells, eosinophils); prominence of Kupffer cells and bile ducts; cholestasis with bile plugs.
Treatment	Supportive care; follow up to determine continued presence of HBsAg for at least 6 months as sign of chronic hepatitis; vaccine available for prevention.
Discussion	**Hepatitis B immune globulin** plus **hepatitis B vaccine** are recommended for parenteral or mucosal exposure to blood and for newborns of HBsAg-positive mothers. The infection is divided into the prodromal, icteric, and convalescent phases; **5% proceed to chronic hepatitis** with increased risk for cirrhosis and **hepatocellular carcinoma**. Unlike hepatitis A, hepatitis B has a long incubation period (3 months). Hepatitis B virus is an enveloped, partially circular DNA virus of the **hepadna** family that contains a DNA-dependent DNA polymerase. The continued presence of HBsAg after infection has clinically resolved indicates a chronic carrier state.
Atlas Links	U̲C̲V̲ M-M1-030

ID/CC	A 30-year-old male is referred for an evaluation of **intermittent jaundice** over the past 2 years.
HPI	He also complains of diarrhea, skin rash, and weight loss. He received a **blood transfusion** 3 years ago, when he was injured in a motorcycle accident. He denies any IV drug use or any history of neuropsychiatric disorders in his family.
PE	**Icterus**; firm, **tender hepatomegaly**; splenomegaly; no evidence of ascites; no Kayser–Fleischer rings found on slit-lamp examination (vs. Wilson's disease).
Labs	Direct hyperbilirubinemia; markedly raised serum transaminase levels; **hepatitis B (HBV) serology negative**; enzyme immunoassay of antibodies to structural and nonstructural enzyme proteins of **hepatitis C** (C200, C33c, C22-3) **positive**.
Micro Pathology	On liver biopsy, presence of ballooning degeneration; fatty changes; **portal inflammation with necrosis of hepatocytes within parenchyma** or immediately adjacent to portal areas ("PIECEMEAL NECROSIS").
Treatment	Ribavirin and α_{2b}-interferon; supportive management.
Discussion	Hepatitis C belongs to the **flavivirus** family and is currently the most important cause of **post-transfusion viral hepatitis**; 90% of cases involve percutaneous transmission. Greater than 50% of cases progress to chronic hepatitis, leading to cirrhosis in 20%.
Atlas Link	UCV1 M-M1-031

HEPATITIS C—CHRONIC ACTIVE

ID/CC A 10-year-old male complains of generalized weakness, faintness on exertion, and occasional epigastric pain.

HPI His mother has noticed that he often **eats soil and other inedible things** (PICA).

PE Pallor; puffy face and dependent edema.

Labs CBC: **microcytic, hypochromic anemia; eosinophilia. Low serum iron and ferritin**; elevated serum transferrin; reduced bone marrow hemosiderin; **hypoproteinemia**; stool exam revealed **eggs of *Ancylostoma duodenale*** (ovoid eggs with thin transparent shell that reveal the segmented embryo within).

Treatment **Albendazole** or mebendazole; **iron supplementation** to treat iron deficiency anemia.

Discussion Infection with hookworms, either *Ancylostoma duodenale* or *Necator americanus*, is more likely where insanitary conditions exist; individuals at risk include children, gardeners, plumbers or electricians who are in contact with soil, and armed-forces personnel. Hookworm eggs excreted in the feces hatch in the soil, releasing larvae that develop into infective larvae. Percutaneous larval penetration is the principal mode of human infection. From the skin, hookworm larvae travel via the bloodstream to the lungs, enter the alveoli, ascend the bronchotracheal tree to the pharynx, and are swallowed. Although transpulmonary larval passage may elicit a transient **eosinophilic pneumonitis** (LÖFFLER'S PNEUMONITIS), this phenomenon is much less common with hookworm infections than with roundworm infections. The major health impact of hookworm infection, however, is iron loss resulting from the 0.1 to 0.4 mL of blood ingested daily by each adult worm. In malnourished hosts, such blood loss can lead to **severe iron deficiency anemia**.

ID/CC	A 14-year-old **malnourished child** died soon after hospitalization due to an **extensive small bowel rupture and shock**.
HPI	He had presented to the emergency room with **massive bloody diarrhea**. His history at admission revealed the presence of abdominal pain, fever, and diarrhea of a few days' duration; his symptoms had developed **after he ate leftover meat** at a fast-food restaurant.
PE	He was dehydrated, pale, and hypotensive at time of admission and developed signs of peritonitis and shock shortly before his death.
Labs	Culture and exam of necrotizing intestinal lesions isolated *Clostridium perfringens* type **C** producing beta toxin.
Gross Pathology	Autopsy revealed ruptured small intestine, mucosal ulcerations, and **gas production** in the wall.
Micro Pathology	Microscopic exam revealed necrosis and acute inflammation in the ileum.
Treatment	Patient died despite aggressive fluid and electrolyte replacement, bowel decompression, and antibiotic therapy (penicillin, clindamycin, or doxycycline); surgery had been planned in view of rupture of the small bowel.
Discussion	Necrotizing enterocolitis is a condition affecting poorly nourished persons who suddenly feast on meat (pigbel). It is associated with *Clostridium perfringens* type **C** and **beta enterotoxin**; beta toxin paralyzes the villi and causes friability and necrosis of the bowel wall. Immunization of children in New Guinea with beta-toxoid vaccine has dramatically decreased the incidence of the disease.
Atlas Links	<u>UCVI</u> M-M1-033A, M-M1-033B, PG-M1-033

NECROTIZING ENTEROCOLITIS

ID/CC	A 7-year-old male who has been hospitalized for treatment of **acute lymphocytic leukemia** complains of **copious watery diarrhea**, right lower quadrant **abdominal pain**, and **fever**.
HPI	He was diagnosed as **neutropenic** (due to aggressive cytotoxic chemotherapy) a few days ago.
PE	VS: fever; tachycardia; tachypnea. PE: pallor; sternal tenderness; axillary lymphadenopathy; hepatosplenomegaly; abdominal distention; moderate dehydration.
Labs	CBC: severe **neutropenia**; anemia; thrombocytopenia. PBS and bone marrow studies suggest he is in remission; blood culture grows *Clostridium septicum*.
Imaging	CT, abdomen: **thickening of cecal wall**.
Gross Pathology	Mucosal ulcers and inflammation in **ileocecal region** of small intestine.
Treatment	Aggressive **supportive measures**; surgical intervention; appropriate **antibiotics** (penicillin G, ampicillin, or clindamycin).
Discussion	Neutropenic enterocolitis is a fulminant form of necrotizing enteritis that occurs in neutropenic patients; neutropenia is often related to cyclic neutropenia, leukemia, aplastic anemia, or chemotherapy. In postmortem exams of patients who have died of leukemia, infections of the cecal area (TYPHLITIS) are frequently found; *Clostridium septicum* is the most common organism isolated from the blood of such patients.

ID/CC	A 25-year-old male complains of **midepigastric pain** that usually begins **1 to 2 hours after eating** and occasionally awakens him at night.
HPI	The patient has been diagnosed with **duodenal ulcers** several times in the past, but his **symptoms have** consistently **recurred** even after therapy with H_2 blockers, antacids, and sucralfate.
PE	VS: stable. PE: pallor; epigastric tenderness on deep palpation.
Labs	CBC: normocytic, normochromic anemia. Stool positive for occult blood.
Imaging	UGI: ulcerations in antrum of stomach and duodenum; antral biopsy specimens yield **positive urease test**.
Gross Pathology	Grossly round ulcer (may also be oval) seen as sharply punched-out defect with relatively straight walls and slight overhanging of mucosal margin (heaped-up margin is characteristic of a malignant lesion); smooth and clean ulcer base.
Micro Pathology	No evidence of malignancy; **antral biopsies** reveal presence of **chronic mucosal inflammation**.
Treatment	Triple therapy with amoxicillin, metronidazole, and bismuth subsalicylate; triple therapy with clarithromycin, omeprazole, and tinidazole is now considered effective and relatively free of side effects.
Discussion	*Helicobacter pylori* grows overlying the antral gastric mucosal cells; 40% of healthy individuals and approximately 50% of patients with peptic disease harbor this organism. Although *H. pylori* **does not breach the epithelial barrier**, colonization of the antral mucosal layer by this organism is associated with structural alterations of the gastric mucosa and hence with a high prevalence of antral gastritis. Despite the fact that *H. pylori* does not grow on duodenal mucosa, it is strongly associated with duodenal ulcer, and eradication of the organism in patients with refractory peptic ulcer disease decreases the risk of recurrence.
Atlas Links	UCV1 M-M1-035A, M-M1-035B, M-M1-035C, PG-M1-035

PEPTIC ULCER DISEASE (*H. PYLORI*)

ID/CC A **4-year-old** male is brought to the physician by his parents, who complain that the child has had **intense perianal itching**, especially **during the night**.

HPI The child is otherwise healthy, and his developmental progress is normal.

PE Perianal excoriation noted.

Labs Cellulose adhesive tape secured to perianal area during the night reveals presence of *Enterobius vermicularis* eggs that were **flattened on one side, were embryonated, and had a thick shell**; no parasites found on stool exam.

Treatment Strict **personal hygiene**; drugs used include **albendazole, mebendazole, piperazine**, and **pyrantel pamoate**.

Discussion Infection is caused by *Enterobius vermicularis*. Adult worms are located primarily in the cecal region; **female adult worms migrate to the perianal area during the night and deposit their eggs**. Direct person-to-person **infection occurs by** ingestion and **swallowing of eggs; autoinoculation** occurs by contamination of fingers. The life cycle is completed in about 6 weeks.

ID/CC	A **10-month-old** male presents with fever and severe **vomiting** followed by **watery diarrhea**.
HPI	His stools are loose and watery without blood or mucus.
PE	VS: fever; tachycardia. PE: child is irritable; moderate dehydration.
Labs	Absence of leukocytes on fecal stain; rotavirus detected with **ELISA; electron microscopy** with negative staining identifies **rotavirus** on stool ultrafiltrates.
Micro Pathology	Major histopathologic lesions are characterized by reversible involvement of the proximal small intestine; mucosa remains intact with shortening of villi, a mixed inflammatory infiltration of lamina propria, and hyperplasia of the mucosal crypt cells; electron microscopy reveals distended cisterns of endoplasmic reticulum, mitochondrial swelling, and sparse, irregular microvilli.
Treatment	**Fluid replacement therapy**.
Discussion	Rotavirus group A is the single **most important cause** of endemic, **severe diarrheal illness in infants and young children worldwide**; it occurs with greater frequency during winter months in temperate climates and during the dry season in tropical climates. In the United States, rotavirus accounts for 50% of all childhood diarrheas, has an incubation period of 48 hours, is transmitted by the fecal-oral route, and lasts only a few days. Some children subsequently develop lactose intolerance, which lasts for a few weeks.

ROTAVIRUS DIARRHEA IN INFANTS

ID/CC	A 30-year-old male presents with sudden-onset, crampy **abdominal pain and diarrhea**.
HPI	The diarrhea is **watery** and contains **mucus**. The patient also complains of low-grade fever with chills, malaise, nausea, and vomiting. Careful history reveals that he had ingested **partially cooked eggs** at a poultry farm 24 hours before his symptoms began.
PE	VS: fever; tachycardia. PE: mild diffuse abdominal tenderness; mild dehydration.
Labs	Stool culture yields *Salmonella typhimurium*; stained stool demonstrates PMNs.
Gross Pathology	Intestinal mucosal erythema (limited to the colon) and some superficial ulcers.
Micro Pathology	Mixed inflammatory infiltrate in mucosa; superficial epithelial erosions.
Treatment	Fluid and electrolyte replacement therapy; **antibiotics withheld**, as they **prolong carrier state**. Antibiotic therapy only for malnourished, severely ill, bacteremic, and sickle cell disease patients.
Discussion	Salmonella infection is acquired through the ingestion of food (**eggs, meat, poultry**) or water contaminated with animal or human feces; individuals with **low gastric acidity** are also susceptible.

ID/CC	A 50-year-old alcoholic white male presents with **fever, abdominal pain**, and rapidly progressive distention of the abdomen.
HPI	He was diagnosed with **alcoholic cirrhosis** 1 month ago, when he was admitted to the hospital with jaundice and hematemesis.
PE	VS: fever. PE: icterus; on palpation, abdominal tenderness with guarding; fluid thrill and shifting dullness to percussion (due to **ascites**); **splenomegaly**; decreased bowel sounds.
Labs	CBC: **leukocytosis**. Ascitic fluid leukocyte count > 500/cc; PMNs (350/cc) elevated; ascitic proteins and glucose depressed; gram-negative bacilli in ascitic fluid; *Escherichia coli* isolated in culture; elevated AST and ALT (AST > ALT).
Imaging	KUB: ground-glass haziness (due to ascites); no evidence of free air. US, abdomen: cirrhotic shrunken liver; **ascites; splenomegaly; increased portal vein diameter and flow**. EGD: esophageal varices.
Gross Pathology	Fibrinopurulent exudate covering surface of peritoneum; fibrosis may lead to formation of adhesions.
Micro Pathology	PMNs and fibrin on serosal surfaces in various stages with presence of granulation tissue and fibrosis.
Treatment	Specific organism-sensitive antibiotics or empiric therapy (such as cefotaxime or β-lactamase-resistant penicillin) for gram-negative aerobic bacilli and gram-positive cocci; supportive treatment for cirrhosis.
Discussion	The spontaneous or primary form of peritonitis occurs in patients with advanced chronic liver disease and concomitant ascites; *E. coli* is the most common cause of secondary peritonitis.

SPONTANEOUS BACTERIAL PERITONITIS

ID/CC	A 25-year-old male U.S. citizen on **vacation in Mexico** presents with abrupt-onset explosive **watery diarrhea, abdominal cramps**, and a **low-grade fever** and chills.
HPI	The patient does not complain of tenesmus or passage of blood or mucus in his stools, but he does complain of a feeling of **urgency** to defecate.
PE	VS: low-grade fever. PE: unremarkable.
Labs	No erythrocytes, WBCs, or parasites seen in stained stool; bioassays for enterotoxigenic *Escherichia coli* (**ETEC**) reveal presence of the labile **enterotoxin (LT)** (tests available only for research purposes).
Treatment	Fluid replacement; antibiotics (fluoroquinolone or TMP-SMX) with loperamide; prevention with careful hygienic practices and prophylactic fluoroquinolone or bismuth subsalicylate with loperamide.
Discussion	Traveler's diarrhea is a self-limited condition that develops within 1 to 2 days of ingestion of contaminated food or drinks. Over three-fourths of cases of traveler's diarrhea are caused by bacteria, with enterotoxigenic *E. coli* the most frequent cause (may also be caused by enteropathogenic *E. coli* and, in Mexico, by an enteroadherent *E. coli*). Other common pathogens include *Shigella* species, *Campylobacter jejuni, Aeromonas* species, *Plesiomonas shigelloides, Salmonella* species, and noncholera vibrios. Rotavirus and Norwalk agent are the most common viral causes; *Giardia, Cryptosporidium*, and, rarely, *Entamoeba histolytica* are parasitic pathogens. Enterotoxigenic *E. coli* produce enterotoxins that bind to intestinal receptors and **activate adenyl cyclase** in the intestinal cell to produce an increase in the level of the cyclic nucleotides cAMP (LT, labile toxin) and cGMP (ST, stable toxin), which markedly augments sodium, chloride, and water loss, thereby producing a **secretory diarrhea**.

ID/CC A 30-year-old male presents with sudden-onset fever, colicky **abdominal pain**, and **watery diarrhea**.

HPI He had eaten **raw oysters** at a friend's party the day before (incubation period 4 hours to 4 days).

PE VS: fever; tachycardia. PE: no dehydration; diffuse abdominal tenderness; increased bowel sounds.

Labs *Vibrio parahaemolyticus* isolated from stool in a high-salt-content (halophilic vibrio) culture medium; PMNs in stool; **Kanagawa phenomenon** (beta-hemolysis on medium containing human blood; done as an indicator for pathogenicity) **positive**.

Treatment Fluid and electrolyte balance; antibiotics not required (since they do not shorten course of infection).

Discussion **Seafood** is the main source of the organism. After ingestion, *Vibrio parahaemolyticus* multiplies in the gut and produces a **diarrheal enterotoxin**.

41 *VIBRIO PARAHAEMOLYTICUS* FOOD POISONING

ID/CC A 35-year-old male presents to the emergency room with high-grade fever, marked weakness, and a hemorrhagic **vesiculobullous skin eruption**.

HPI He had just returned from deep-sea fishing in the Gulf of Mexico, where he had consumed large quantities of **seafood**. He has been diagnosed with **chronic liver disease** (due to hemochromatosis).

PE VS: fever; hypotension; tachycardia. PE: icterus; vesiculobullous skin lesions seen on an otherwise-bronzed complexion.

Labs Blood culture on **high-salt medium** (halophilic bacteria) reveals growth of *Vibrio vulnificus*; evidence of hemochromatosis (hyperglycemia, hyperbilirubinemia, increased serum iron).

Treatment **Ceftazidime** and **doxycycline, ciprofloxacin**; supportive.

Discussion Halophilic *Vibrio vulnificus* should be suspected and treated in any individual with chronic liver disease who presents with septicemia and skin lesions 1 to 3 days following seafood ingestion.

VIBRIO VULNIFICUS **FOOD POISONING**

ID/CC	A 56-year-old white male complains of **diarrhea** and bloating for **several months** along with ankle swelling.
HPI	He also complains of memory loss, fever, **arthritis** in the knees and hands, and **weight loss**.
PE	VS: fever. PE: thin, gaunt male; muscle wasting; swollen, tender right wrist and ankle; axillary and femoral lymphadenopathy; ecchymoses of chest and arms.
Labs	CBC/PBS: macrocytic, hypochromic anemia; hypoalbuminemia; **increased fecal fat** (steatorrhea).
Imaging	UGI/SBFT: nonspecific dilatation of small bowel.
Gross Pathology	Atrophy of intestinal mucosa; inflammatory infiltrate in synovia of joints.
Micro Pathology	Small bowel biopsy reveals **characteristic macrophages** containing bacilli with **PAS** reagent staining; characteristic gram-negative actinomycete bacilli in macrophages, PMNs, and epithelial cells of lamina propria; dilated lymphatics; flattening of intestinal villi.
Treatment	Bactrim (TMP-SMX) or ceftriaxone for 1 year.
Discussion	Caused by infection with *Tropheryma whippelii*; produces **malabsorption** of fat-soluble vitamins, protein, iron, folic acid, and vitamin B_{12}.

WHIPPLE'S DISEASE

ID/CC A 28-year-old female complains of **painful swelling of both knees** and **tender skin eruptions** on both shins.

HPI For the past 2 weeks she has also had **watery diarrhea** that developed after she consumed some **raw pork**. She also complains of low-grade fever and mild abdominal pain.

PE VS: low-grade fever; tachycardia. PE: mild dehydration; swollen and warm knee joints with painful restriction of all movements (ARTHRITIS); multiple **tender, erythematous plaques and nodules** (ERYTHEMA NODOSUM) seen over both shins.

Labs CBC: leukocytosis. *Yersinia enterocolitica* isolated from stool; patient is **HLA-B27 positive**.

Micro Pathology Oval ulcers with long axis in the direction of bowel flow, similar to ulcers caused by typhoid fever (intestinal tubercular ulcers are transverse).

Treatment Supportive; antibiotics (aminoglycosides, fluoroquinolones) indicated in severe infections.

Discussion *Yersinia enterocolitica* is an invasive gram-negative **intracellular pathogen** that causes **gastroenteritis**, most frequently involving the distal ileum and colon (enterotoxin mediated), **mesenteric adenitis** (due to necrotizing and suppurative gut lesions) and ileitis **(pseudoappendicitis)**, and sepsis; infection may trigger a variety of **autoimmune phenomena**, including erythema nodosum, reactive arthritis, and possibly Graves' disease, especially in HLA-B27-positive individuals. Spread is by the fecal-oral route and occurs via contaminated milk products or water, swine, or household pet feces.

ID/CC	A 3-year-old **albino** male is referred to a specialist for an evaluation of a suspected immune deficiency.
HPI	His parents report **recurrent** respiratory, skin, and oral **infections with gram-negative and gram-positive** organisms. He also has a history of bruising easily.
PE	**Partial albinism**; light-brown hair with silvery tint; **nystagmus; photophobia** on eye reflex exam; chronic gingivitis and periodontitis; purpuric patches over areas of repeated minimal trauma; mild hepatomegaly; no lymphadenopathy.
Labs	CBC/PBS: **decreased neutrophil count** with normal platelet count; **large cytoplasmic granules** (GIANT LYSOSOMES) in WBCs on Wright-stained peripheral blood smears. Prolonged bleeding time; impaired platelet aggregation; normal clotting time and PTT; normal nitroblue tetrazolium test.
Treatment	Largely supportive; ascorbic acid, prophylactic antibiotics, acyclovir.
Discussion	Chédiak–Higashi syndrome is an **autosomal-recessive** disorder that is due to a **defect in polymerization of microtubules in leukocytes** that causes impairment of chemotaxis, phagocytosis, and formation of phagolysosomes. Patients with this disorder usually present with **recurrent pyogenic staphylococcal and streptococcal infections**.

CHÉDIAK–HIGASHI SYNDROME

ID/CC	An **8-year-old child** with **sickle cell anemia** is seen with complaints of sudden-onset **pallor of the skin** and mucous membranes, fatigue, and malaise.
HPI	The child suffered a **mild prodromal illness** before developing severe pallor.
PE	VS: no fever; tachycardia; tachypnea; BP normal. PE: severe pallor; mild icterus; no lymphadenopathy, splenomegaly, or hepatomegaly noted.
Labs	CBC: **severe anemia** (Hb 2 g/dL); **reduced leukocyte** and platelet counts; mild hyperbilirubinemia; **absent reticulocytes** and sickled RBCs on peripheral blood smear.
Micro Pathology	Bone marrow biopsy reveals increased numbers of **giant pronormoblasts** (diagnostic of parvovirus infection).
Treatment	Blood transfusions to tide over the crises. Spontaneous recovery in 1 to 2 weeks.
Discussion	Parvovirus infection is the cause of **transient aplastic crises** (may also be due to folic acid deficiency) that occur in patients who have severe **hemolytic disorders**; cessation of erythropoiesis for about 10 days in a normal adult as a result of parvovirus infection would produce a 10% drop in hemoglobin concentration (i.e., a fall of 1% daily would lead to a decline in hemoglobin concentration of 1 to 2 g/dL after 10 days). A patient with severe hemolysis in whom the bone marrow is turning over at a rate seven times normal would experience a 70% decrease in hemoglobin concentration (i.e., a drop from 10 g/dL to 3 g/dL) as a result of a 10-day cessation of erythropoiesis. Although parvovirus can affect all precursor cells, the red cell precursors are most profoundly affected.
Atlas Link	UCV1 H-M1-046

ID/CC	A 35-year-old **Finnish** man complains of **easy fatigability and shortness of breath**.
HPI	He often eats **undercooked or raw freshwater fish**. He also reports vague digestive disturbances such as anorexia, heartburn, and nausea.
PE	PE: pallor.
Labs	CBC/PBS: **megaloblastic anemia**. Blood **vitamin B$_{12}$ levels low**; stool exam reveals presence of **operculated eggs and proglottids of *Diphyllobothrium latum*.**
Treatment	**Niclosamide** or praziquantel.
Discussion	*Diphyllobothrium latum* (fish tapeworm) infection is found in cold climates where **raw or undercooked fish** are eaten. The adult worm attaches to the human jejunum and **competes for absorption of vitamin B$_{12}$**, producing a deficiency that resembles pernicious anemia. Prevention includes proper preparation of fish.

ANEMIA—*DIPHYLLOBOTHRIUM LATUM*

ID/CC A 45-year-old male with refractory **acute myeloid leukemia** who underwent a **bone marrow transplant** from a nonidentical donor presents with an **extensive skin rash**, severe **diarrhea**, and **jaundice**.

HPI Prior to the transplant, which occurred 2 months ago, he **received preparative chemotherapy and radiotherapy** along with broad-spectrum antibiotics. Engraftment was confirmed within 4 weeks by rising leukocyte counts.

PE VS: BP normal. PE: patient is cachectic and moderately dehydrated; icterus noted; violaceous, scaly macules and erythematous papules **resembling lichen planus** seen over extremities.

Labs CBC: falling blood counts; relative eosinophilia. Elevated direct serum bilirubin and transaminases; stool exam reveals no infectious etiology; skin biopsy taken.

Gross Pathology Skin biopsy specimens reveal vacuolar changes of basal cell layer with perivenular lymphocytic infiltrates (CD8+ T cells).

Treatment **High-dose cyclosporine therapy**, rabbit anti-thymocyte globulin, methylprednisolone or anti-T-cell monoclonal antibodies.

Discussion Approximately 30% of bone marrow transplant recipients develop graft-versus-host disease (GVHD). This attack is primarily launched by immunocompetent T lymphocytes derived from the donor's marrow against the cells and tissues of the recipient, which it recognizes as foreign. Cyclosporin A is effective for prevention of GVHD.

ID/CC	A 20-year-old male presents with an extensive **purpuric skin rash, oliguria**, and marked weakness; he also complains of **bloody diarrhea** of 1 week's duration.
HPI	The patient ate **a hamburger** at a fast-food restaurant 2 to 3 **days prior to the onset** of his diarrhea. He has no associated fever.
PE	VS: no fever. PE: dehydration; pallor; extensive purpuric skin rash.
Labs	Stool examination reveals presence of RBCs but **no inflammatory cells** or parasites; culture isolates sorbitol-negative *Escherichia coli*; serotyping studies and effect on HeLa cell culture reveal presence of **enterohemorrhagic *E. coli*** (EHEC) **serotype O157:H7**; elevated BUN and creatinine. CBC/PBS: **microangiopathic anemia** and thrombocytopenia. PT, PTT normal.
Imaging	Sigmoidoscopy: moderately hyperemic mucosa with no evidence of any ulceration.
Micro Pathology	Pathology localized to kidney, where hyaline **thrombi** were seen **in afferent arterioles** and glomerular capillaries.
Treatment	Dialysis and blood transfusion for management of HUS; fluid and electrolyte maintenance; antimicrobial therapy. Most patients who develop HUS as a complication of *E. coli* hemorrhagic colitis die as a result of hemorrhagic complications.
Discussion	Hemorrhagic colitis associated with a Shiga-like toxin producing **EHEC O157:H7** is characterized by grossly bloody diarrhea with remarkably little fever or inflammatory exudate in stool; a significant number of patients develop potentially fatal HUS. EHEC infections can be largely **prevented through adequate cooking of beef**, especially hamburgers.
Atlas Link	UCV1 H-M1-049

HEMOLYTIC-UREMIC SYNDROME (HUS)

ID/CC	A 34-year-old male presents to his primary care physician with a hard, red, painless **swelling** on his left **mandible** that has slowly been growing over the past few weeks and has now begun to **drain pus**.
HPI	The patient **recently had a tooth extraction**.
PE	No acute distress; no other significant findings.
Labs	Gram stain of exudate reveals **branching gram-positive filaments** and characteristic **"sulfur granules"**; non-acid-fast and anaerobic (distinguishes actinomyces from *Nocardia*).
Imaging	XR: no bony destruction.
Gross Pathology	**Sinus tracts** from region of infection to surface with granular exudate.
Micro Pathology	Granulation tissue and fibrosis surrounding a central suppurative necrosis; granulation tissue may also enclose foamy histiocytes and plasma cells.
Treatment	Ampicillin followed by amoxicillin or penicillin G followed by oral penicillin V and, if necessary, surgical drainage and removal of necrotic tissue.
Discussion	*Actinomyces israelii* is a part of the normal flora of the mouth (crypts of tonsils and tartar of teeth), so most patients have a history of surgery or trauma. There is **no person-to-person spread**. Actinomycosis is a chronic suppurative infection and can also involve the abdomen or lungs, especially following a penetrating trauma such as a bullet wound or an intestinal perforation. Pelvic disease is associated with IUD use. Spread occurs contiguously, not hematogenously.
Atlas Link	⬜🅄🅒🅥🅈 M-M1-050

ID/CC A **7-month-old** girl is brought to the pediatric clinic with **wheezing**, respiratory difficulty, and nasal congestion of 3 hours' duration.

HPI She has had rhinorrhea, fever, and cough and had been sneezing for 2 days prior to her visit to the clinic.

PE VS: **tachypnea**. PE: **nasal flaring**; mild central **cyanosis**; accessory muscle use during respiration; hyperexpansion of chest; expiratory and inspiratory wheezes; **rhonchi** over both lung fields.

Labs CBC/PBS: relative **lymphocytosis**. ABGs: **hypoxemia with mild hypercapnia. Respiratory syncytial virus (RSV)** demonstrated on viral culture of throat swab.

Imaging CXR: **hyperinflation**; segmental **atelectasis; interstitial infiltrates**.

Micro Pathology Severe bronchiolitis produces bronchiolar epithelial necrosis, lymphocytic infiltrate, and alveolar exudates.

Treatment Humidified oxygen, bronchodilators, aerosolized **ribavirin**.

Discussion **RSV is the most common cause of bronchiolitis in infants** under 2 years of age; other viral causes include parainfluenza, influenza, and adenovirus. RSV shedding may last 2 or more weeks in children.

ID/CC	An **8-year-old** female presents with pain and swelling of her knee joints, elbows, and lower limbs along with **fever** for the past 2 weeks; she also complains of shortness of breath (DYSPNEA) on exertion.
HPI	The patient had a **sore throat 2 weeks ago**.
PE	VS: fever. PE: **blanching, ring-shaped erythematous rash over trunk and proximal extremities** (ERYTHEMA MARGINATUM); **subcutaneous nodules** at occiput and below extensor tendons in elbow; **swelling with redness of both knee joints and elbows** (POLYARTHRITIS); painfully restricted movement; pedal edema; increased JVP; high-frequency apical systolic murmur with radiation to axillae **(mitral valve insufficiency due to carditis)**; bilateral fine inspiratory basal crepitant rales; mild, tender hepatomegaly.
Labs	CBC: leukocytosis. *Streptococcus pyogenes* on throat swab; markedly **elevated ASO titers; elevated ESR; elevated C-reactive protein (CRP)**; negative blood culture. ECG: **prolonged P-R interval**.
Imaging	CXR: cardiomegaly; increased pulmonary vascular markings. Echo: vegetations over mitral valve with regurgitation.
Gross Pathology	Acute form characterized by **endo-, myo-, and pericarditis** (PANCARDITIS); chronic form characterized by fibrous scarring with calcification and mitral stenosis with verrucous fibrin deposits.
Micro Pathology	Myocardial muscle fiber necrosis enmeshed in collagen; characteristic finding is fibrinoid necrosis surrounded by **perivascular accumulation of mononuclear inflammatory cells** (ASCHOFF CELLS).
Treatment	Aspirin, corticosteroids, and diuretics; penicillin or erythromycin.
Discussion	Acute rheumatic fever is a sequela of upper respiratory infection with group A, β-hemolytic streptococcus; it causes **autoimmune** damage to several organs, primarily the heart. The systemic effects of acute rheumatic fever are immune mediated and are secondary to cross-reactivity of host antistreptococcal antibodies.
Atlas Link	UCV1 M-M1-052

ID/CC A 48-year-old missionary who has lived in Cameroon, **West Africa**, for 20 years is airlifted home because of **lethargy, nuchal rigidity, persistent headache, and drowsiness** that have not responded to antibiotics and supportive treatment.

HPI He states that over the years he has been bitten in the neck several times by a mutumutu, or **tsetse fly** (*GLOSSINA PALPALIS*). He has also had intermittent, generalized erythematous rashes accompanied by fever.

PE Alert but somewhat **incoherent and confused**; sometimes delusional; nuchal rigidity and **tremors of face and lips**; splenomegaly; generalized **rubbery, painless lymphadenopathy**, predominantly in posterior neck and supraclavicular areas (WINTERBOTTOM'S SIGN).

Labs PBS/LP: hypercellular, **trypanosomal** forms present; lymphocytes in CSF. **Elevated IgM**.

Gross Pathology Chancre with erythema and induration at bite site; chancre resolves spontaneously; spleen and lymph nodes enlarged during systemic stage; leptomeninges enlarged during CNS involvement.

Micro Pathology Skin: edema, mononuclear cell inflammation, organisms, and endothelial proliferation; spleen and lymph nodes: histiocytic hyperplasia; CNS: mononuclear cell meningoencephalitis.

Treatment Suramin; pentamidine or eflornithine.

Discussion Also called **sleeping sickness**, African trypanosomiasis is a systemic febrile disease endemic to Africa whose chronic form causes a meningoencephalitis. It is caused by the flagellated protozoans *Trypanosoma brucei gambiense* (West African) and *Trypanosoma brucei rhodesiense* (East African), which are transmitted by the tsetse fly.

ID/CC	A 28-year-old **male homosexual** complains of continuous low-grade **fever, weight loss**, and **diarrhea** of 1 month's duration.
HPI	He also complains of an **extensive skin rash, mucous membrane eruptions, recurrent herpes zoster infection**, and **oral ulcerations**. He reports practicing receptive anal intercourse.
PE	VS: low-grade fever. PS: cachectic; **generalized lymphadenopathy**; maculopapular rash; severe **seborrheic dermatitis; aphthous ulcers**; white confluent patch with corrugated surface (ORAL HAIRY LEUKOPLAKIA) along lateral borders of tongue; **penile warts** (CONDYLOMATA ACUMINATA); extensive multiple pruritic, pink, umbilicated papules 2 to 5 mm in diameter (MOLLUSCUM CONTAGIOSUM).
Labs	CBC: anemia; leukopenia with lymphopenia; thrombocytopenia. **Low CD4+ count**; elevated CD8+ T-cell count; ELISA for HIV-1 positive; **Western blot confirmatory; PCR for viral RNA** (investigation of choice in window period) **positive**.
Micro Pathology	**Oral hairy leukoplakia**; lesions show keratin projections resembling hairs, koilocytosis, and little atypia; hybridization techniques reveal **Epstein–Barr virus** in lesions.
Treatment	Prophylactic antibiotics for prevention of opportunistic infections while monitoring CD4+ T-cell counts; antiretroviral drugs (zidovudine, didanosine, zalcitabine, and protease inhibitors); counseling and rehabilitative measures.
Discussion	AIDS-related complex (ARC) consists of symptomatic conditions in an HIV-infected patient that are not included in the AIDS surveillance case definition and that meet at least one of the following criteria: (1) the conditions are indicative of a defect in cell-mediated immunity; or (2) the conditions have a clinical course or management that is complicated by HIV infection.
Atlas Link	UCV2 Z-M1-054

ID/CC A 28-year-old male from **India** complains of gradual-onset, intermittent, **crampy abdominal pain** with one to four **foul-smelling, frothy loose stools daily**.

HPI His stools sometimes contain blood and mucus. He also complains of flatulence, tenesmus, and, at times, alternating diarrhea and constipation.

PE Slight tenderness during palpation of cecum and ascending colon; no hepatomegaly.

Labs CBC: mild leukocytosis; no eosinophilia. Fresh stool examination reveals presence of *Entamoeba histolytica* **cysts and motile hematophagous trophozoites**; serology for antiamebic antibodies is positive.

Imaging Colonoscopy: **multiple colonic mucosal ulcers** that are slightly raised and covered with shaggy exudate; mucosa between ulcers normal.

Micro Pathology Biopsy specimens reveal lesions extending under adjacent intact mucosa to produce classical **"flask-shaped" ulcers**; amebic trophozoites demonstrated at base of ulcer.

Treatment **Metronidazole** (drug of choice) followed by paromomycin or iodoquinol.

Discussion *Entamoeba histolytica* cysts are infective and are transmitted through contaminated water, raw vegetables, food handlers, and fecal-oral or oral-anal contact. The sites of involvement, in order of frequency, are the cecum and ascending colon, rectum, sigmoid colon, appendix, and terminal ileum. Trophozoites are the invasive form of the organism, causing colitis or distant infection by hematogenous spread. Complications include perforation of the bowel; liver abscess with pleural, pericardial, or peritoneal rupture; bowel obstruction by ameboma; and skin ulcers around the perineum and genitalia.

Atlas Link UCV1 M-M1-055

ID/CC	A 45-year-old male Peace Corps volunteer who recently spent 2 years in rural Mexico complains of a **spiking fever**, malaise, headache, and **right upper quadrant abdominal pain**.
HPI	He admits to having had **bloody diarrhea with mucus** (DYSENTERY) and tenesmus that disappeared with some pills that he took several months ago.
PE	VS: fever (39.6°C). PE: pallor; slight jaundice; tender 3+ **hepatomegaly** with no rebound tenderness; pain on fist percussion of right lower ribs.
Labs	CBC: leukocytosis with neutrophilia. Amebic cysts in stool specimen (not concurrent with abscess); positive serology for antibodies to *Entamoeba histolytica*.
Imaging	CXR: elevation of right hemidiaphragm; small right pleural effusion. CT/US: cavitating lesion in **right lobe of liver** (due to abscess).
Gross Pathology	Multiple colonic mucosal ulcers, slightly raised and covered with shaggy exudate; enlarged liver with **one large abscess** on right lobe containing chocolate-colored pus; abscess may rupture and spread to lungs, brain, or other organs.
Micro Pathology	Sterile pus; ameba may be obtained from periphery of lesion.
Treatment	Metronidazole; needle evacuation; surgery in case of treatment failure or rupture.
Discussion	Prior travel to endemic areas plus a triad of fever, hepatomegaly, and right upper quadrant pain are hallmarks of hepatic liver abscess. Colitis precedes the liver abscess; amebas then invade the gut wall and enter portal circulation.

AMEBIC LIVER ABSCESS

ID/CC A **15-year-old male** who resides in Florida presents with **nausea** and vomiting, **fever**, and **marked neck stiffness**.

HPI He also complains of a severe bifrontal headache. Careful history reveals that he **swam for several hours in brackish water** approximately a week ago.

PE VS: fever; tachycardia. PE: signs of meningeal irritation (neck rigidity, positive Kernig's sign and Brudzinski's sign); funduscopy reveals mild papilledema.

Labs LP: bloody CSF (raised RBC count may also be due to examiner's inability to recognize proliferating amebas) shows intense neutrophilia, pleocytosis, high protein, and low sugar; no organism seen on Gram, ZN, or India ink staining of CSF; **wet preparation** of CSF reveals viable *Naegleria* **trophozoites**; diagnosis confirmed using direct fluorescent antibody staining.

Gross Pathology Lesions are mostly present in the olfactory nerves and brain. Focal hemorrhages, extensive fibrinoid necrosis, and blood vessel thrombosis with nerve tissue necrosis.

Micro Pathology *Naegleria fowleri* trophozoites seen as 10- to 20-μm-diameter organisms with large nucleus, small granular cytoplasm, distinct ectoplasm, and bulbous pseudopodia.

Treatment Intracisternal and IV **amphotericin B**, miconazole, rifampin; prognosis is very poor.

Discussion Primary amebic meningoencephalitis is caused by amebas of the genus *Naegleria* or *Acanthamoeba*. The former most often affects children and young adults, appears to be acquired by swimming in warm, fresh/brackish water, and is almost always fatal, with the ameba gaining entry into the arachnoid space through the nasal cribriform plate. *Acanthamoeba* infections involve older, immunocompromised individuals and are sometimes characterized by spontaneous recovery.

ID/CC	A 30-year-old male goes to the emergency room because of **dyspnea**, cyanosis, hemoptysis, and chest pain.
HPI	He has had a high fever, malaise, and a **nonproductive cough** for 1 week. The patient is a **sheep farmer** who remembers having been treated for **dark black skin lesions** in the past.
PE	VS: fever. PE: dyspnea; cyanosis; bilateral rales heard over lungs.
Labs	CBC: normal. Negative blood and sputum cultures; diagnosis of anthrax confirmed by fourfold increase in indirect microhemagglutination titer.
Imaging	CXR: mediastinal widening. CT, chest: evidence of **"hemorrhagic mediastinitis."**
Gross Pathology	Patchy consolidation; vesicular papules covered by **black eschar**.
Micro Pathology	Lungs show fibrinous exudate with many organisms but few PMNs.
Treatment	Isolate and treat with IV penicillin G or ciprofloxacin.
Discussion	Anthrax is caused by infection with *Bacillus anthracis*. A cell-free anthrax vaccine is available to protect those employed in industries associated with a high risk of anthrax transmission (farmers, veterinarians, tannery or wool workers).

ID/CC A 38-year-old male receiving cytotoxic **chemotherapy** (immunosuppressed) for acute leukemia presents with **pleuritic chest pain**, hemoptysis, **fever**, and chills.

HPI He also complains of dyspnea, tachypnea, and a **productive cough**.

PE VS: fever. PE: severe respiratory distress; bilateral rales heard over lungs.

Labs CBC: severe **neutropenia**. Negative blood and sputum culture for bacteria.

Imaging CXR: necrotizing bronchopneumonia.

Gross Pathology **Necrotizing bronchopneumonia**; abscesses.

Micro Pathology Lung biopsy identifies *Aspergillus* with septate, acutely branching hyphae (visualized by silver stains); necrotizing inflammation; vascular thrombi with hyphae (due to **blood vessel invasion**).

Treatment IV amphotericin B or itraconazole.

Discussion The most lethal form of infection, invasive aspergillosis, is seen primarily in severely immunocompromised individuals, i.e., patients with **AIDS**; patients with prolonged, **severe neutropenia** following cytotoxic chemotherapy; patients with **chronic granulomatous disease**; and patients receiving **glucocorticoids** and other **immunosuppressive drugs** (e.g., transplant recipients).

Atlas Links ⬚ⓤⒸⓋⓘ⬚ M-M1-059A, M-M1-059B, M-M1-059C

ID/CC A 50-year-old male presents to the ER with complaints of **recurrent**, sudden-onset, **severe breathlessness**, wheezing, fever, chills, and a **productive cough** (sometimes producing **brown bronchial casts**).

HPI The patient has had steroid-dependent **chronic bronchial asthma** for many years and has no history of foreign travel or contact with a TB patient. He has a history of **occasional hemoptysis**.

PE VS: fever; marked tachycardia; severe tachypnea. PE: respiratory distress; central cyanosis; wheezing; rhonchi and coarse rales over both lung fields.

Labs CBC: **eosinophilia**. Oxygen saturation low. Very high titers of specific **IgE antibodies against** *Aspergillus* present (specific marker for the disease); sputum cultures positive for *Aspergillus*; **skin tests** to *Aspergillus* antigens **positive**. PFTs: obstructive picture (due to underlying asthma).

Imaging CXR: **segmental infiltrate** in upper lobes (these infiltrates are segmental because they correspond directly to the affected bronchi); **branching, fingerlike shadows** from mucoid impaction of dilated central bronchi (virtually **pathognomonic** of allergic bronchopulmonary aspergillosis). CT, chest: evidence of **proximal bronchiectasis**.

Treatment Oral corticosteroids or beclomethasone.

Discussion Allergic bronchopulmonary aspergillosis (ABPA) is a hypersensitivity disorder that primarily affects the central bronchi; immediate and Arthus-type hypersensitivity reactions are involved in its pathogenesis. The onset of the disease occurs most often in the fourth and fifth decades, and virtually all patients have long-standing atopic asthma. Untreated ABPA leads to proximal bronchiectasis.

ID/CC A 50-year-old **alcoholic male** presents with a high-grade **fever, cough, copious, foul-smelling sputum**, and pleuritic right-sided chest pain.

HPI His wife reports that he was brought home in a **semiconscious state a few days ago**, when he was found lying on the roadside heavily under the influence of alcohol.

PE VS: fever. PE: signs of consolidation elicited over **right middle and lower pulmonary lobes**.

Labs Sputum reveals abundant PMN leukocytes and mixed oral flora; **culture yields _Bacteroides melaninogenicus (Prevotella melaninogenica)_ and other _Bacteroides_ species, _Fusobacterium_, microaerophilic streptococci**, and _Peptostreptococcus_.

Imaging CXR: **consolidation involving apical segment of right lower lobe and posterior segments of middle lobe**; large cavity with air-fluid level (ABSCESS) also seen.

Treatment **Clindamycin**.

Discussion Alcoholism, drug abuse, administration of sedatives or anesthesia, head trauma, and seizures or other neurologic disorders are most often responsible for the development of aspiration pneumonia. Because anaerobes are the dominant flora of the upper GI tract (outnumbering aerobic or facultative bacteria by 10 to 1), they are the dominant organisms in aspiration pneumonia; of particular importance are _Bacteroides melaninogenicus_ (_Prevotella melaninogenica_) and other _Bacteroides_ species (slender, pleomorphic, pale gram-negative rods), _Fusobacterium nucleatum_ (slender gram-negative rods with pointed ends), and anaerobic or microaerophilic streptococci and _Peptostreptococcus_ (small gram-positive cocci in chains or clumps).

ASPIRATION PNEUMONIA WITH LUNG ABSCESS

ID/CC	A 38-year-old **HIV-positive** male is admitted to the hospital with **fever, rigors, night sweats, and diarrhea**.
HPI	He reports excessive weight loss over the past few weeks. He was treated for *Pneumocystis* **pneumonia** a few weeks ago and still reports a persistent productive cough.
PE	VS: fever. PE: patient is extremely emaciated; hepatosplenomegaly and lymphadenopathy noted.
Labs	CD4+ count < 50/cc; *Mycobacterium avium-intracellulare* isolated on blood culture; smears of tissues obtained from lymph nodes, bone marrow, spleen, liver, and lungs reveal evidence of acid-fast bacilli, and cultures yield *M. avium*; intestinal infection with *M. avium* proven by culture of stools and colonic biopsy specimens.
Imaging	CT, abdomen: hepatosplenomegaly; retroperitoneal lymphadenopathy; bowel mucosal fold thickening.
Micro Pathology	Despite the presence of many mycobacteria and macrophages, well-formed granulomas were typically absent due to **profound impairment of cell-mediated immunity**.
Treatment	The primary treatment regimen includes clarithromycin and ethambutol with or without rifabutin. The failure rate of therapy is high.
Discussion	*Mycobacterium avium* complex is now the **most frequent opportunistic bacterial infection in patients with AIDS**; it typically occurs late in the course of the syndrome, when other opportunistic infections and neoplasia have already occurred. Prophylaxis against *M. avium-intracellulare* is recommended in AIDS patients with a CD4+ count of < 100/mm^3 (administer azithromycin, clarithromycin, or rifabutin).

ID/CC A 20-year-old male from **India** presents to the ER with **severe nausea and vomiting**.

HPI Careful history reveals that 2 hours ago he ate some **unrefrigerated fried rice** that his wife had cooked the night before. He does not complain of any fever or diarrhea (may or may not be present).

PE VS: no fever. PE: mild dehydration; diffuse mild abdominal tenderness.

Labs Fecal staining reveals no RBCs, WBCs, or parasites; *Bacillus cereus*, **a gram-positive rod**, isolated from vomitus and stool and shown to produce the **emetogenic enterotoxin**.

Treatment Supportive.

Discussion *Bacillus cereus* causes two distinct syndromes: a **diarrheal form** (mediated by an *Escherichia coli* LT-type enterotoxin with an incubation period of 8 to 16 hours; caused by meats and vegetables) and an **emetic form** (mediated by a *Staphylococcus aureus*-type enterotoxin with an incubation period of 1 to 8 hours; caused by fried rice). Proper food handling and refrigeration of boiled rice are largely preventive.

BACILLUS CEREUS FOOD POISONING

ID/CC A 30-year-old male who recently emigrated from **Peru** presents with an extensive **nodular skin eruption**, mild arthralgias, and occasional fever.

HPI One month ago, the patient had a high-grade **fever** that was accompanied by excessive weakness, dyspnea, and passage of **cola-colored urine**; the fever subsided after 2 weeks, but his weakness has progressed since that time.

PE Pallor; mild icterus; extensive skin rash comprising **purplish nodular lesions** of varying sizes seen on face, trunk, and limbs; mild hepatosplenomegaly; funduscopy reveals **retinal hemorrhages**.

Labs **Intraerythrocytic coccobacillary**-form bacteria visible in thick and thin films stained with Giemsa; **bacteria** seen and **isolated from skin lesions**; indirect serum bilirubin elevated. PBS: macrocytic, hypochromic anemia with polychromasia; marked reticulocytosis (due to hemolytic anemia); Coombs' test negative.

Micro Pathology Skin biopsy of vascular skin lesions reveals endothelial proliferation and histiocytic hyperplasia; electron microscopy of verrucous tissue shows *Bartonella bacilliformis* in interstitial tissue.

Treatment **Chloramphenicol, penicillin, erythromycin, norfloxacin**, and **tetracycline** are effective; rifampicin is indicated for treatment of verrucous forms.

Discussion Bartonellosis is a sandfly-borne bacterial disease occurring only on the **western coast of South America** at high altitudes; the causative agent is a motile, pleomorphic bacillus, *Bartonella bacilliformis*. Two stages of the disease are recognized: an **initial febrile stage** associated with a **hemolytic anemia** (OROYA FEVER) and a later cutaneous stage characterized by **hemangiomatous nodules** (VERRUGA PERUANA).

ID/CC   A 32-year-old male is referred to a tertiary care center with **chronic pneumonia** and **warty lesions** on his left upper limb.

HPI   The patient is from the **southeastern United States**. His skin lesions are nonpruritic and painless. He also complains of malaise, weight loss, night sweats, chest pain, breathlessness, and hoarseness.

PE   VS: fever; tachycardia; mild tachypnea. PE: **bilateral rales and rhonchi**; raised, **verrucous, and crusted lesions** with serpiginous border located on left upper extremity; small abscesses demonstrable when superficial crust was removed.

Labs   Sputum and pus from cutaneous lesions demonstrate **spherical cells** (8 to 15 mm in diameter) that have a **thick-walled, refractile double contour** and show unipolar (broad-based) budding; culture of pus and sputum on Sabouraud's agar yields **growth of *Blastomyces***; no evidence of acid-fast bacilli found either on staining or on culture; Gomori's methenamine silver staining of lung tissue does not reveal *Pneumocystis*.

Imaging   CXR: bilateral alveolar consolidations with air bronchograms.

Micro Pathology   Epithelioid macrophages and giant cells surrounding a suppurative center; skin lesions show pseudoepitheliomatous hyperplasia very similar to squamous cell carcinoma.

Treatment   Itraconazole is treatment of choice in most patients; amphotericin B, fluconazole, and ketoconazole are alternative drugs.

Discussion   Blastomycosis is a systemic mycotic infection of humans and dogs that is characterized by suppuration and granulomatous lesions and is caused by the **dimorphic fungus *Blastomyces dermatitidis***; the disease is **endemic in the southeastern and south-central portions of the United States**, and several pockets of infection extend north along the Mississippi and Ohio rivers into central Canada. Clinical disease most commonly involves the lungs (acquired by spore inhalation) and then, by hematogenous dissemination, the skin, the skeletal system, and the male genitourinary tract. Infection cannot be passed from person to person.

Atlas Link   U C V I M-M1-065

ID/CC	A 25-year-old male presents with sudden-onset **double vision** (DIPLOPIA), **dry mouth, weakness, dysarthria**, and **dysphagia**.
HPI	He has no previous history of episodic weakness or of dog or tick bites (vs. myasthenia gravis, rabies, or Lyme disease). Last night, he ate some **home-canned food**.
PE	VS: no fever. PE: patient alert; ptosis; bilateral **third and tenth cranial nerve palsy**; symmetric **flaccid paralysis** of all four limbs; deep tendon reflexes reduced; no sensory loss seen; decreased bowel sounds.
Labs	Botulinum toxin detected in patient's serum and canned-food sample with specific antiserum.
Treatment	Antitoxin; close monitoring of respiratory status; intubation for respiratory failure.
Discussion	The disease is characterized by gradual return of muscle strength in most cases. Botulinum toxin is a zinc metalloprotease that cleaves specific components of synaptic vesicle docking and fusion complexes, thus **inhibiting the release of acetylcholine at the neuromuscular junction**. The disease in adults is due to **ingestion of the toxin** rather than to bacterial infection. Botulism is also seen in infants secondary to the ingestion of *Clostridium botulinum* spores in **honey**.

ID/CC	A 28-year-old white male visits his family doctor complaining of acute **pain in both hip joints** together with weakness, backache, myalgias, arthralgias, and **undulating fever** of **2 months' duration**; this morning he woke up with pain in his right testicle.
HPI	For the past 3 years he has worked at the largest dairy farm in his state. He enjoys **drinking "crude" milk**.
PE	VS: fever. PE: pallor; marked pain on palpation of sacroiliac joints; mild splenomegaly; generalized lymphadenopathy.
Labs	CBC: relative lymphocytosis with normal WBC count. Positive agglutination titer (> 1:160); rising serologic titer over time; small gram-negative rod *Brucella abortus* on blood culture.
Imaging	XR, hips: joint effusion and soft tissue swelling without destruction. MR, spine: evidence of spondylitis.
Gross Pathology	Lymphadenopathy and splenomegaly; hepatomegaly rare.
Micro Pathology	Granulomatous foci in spleen, liver, and lymph nodes, with proliferation of macrophages; epithelioid and giant cells may be seen.
Treatment	Combination therapy with doxycycline or TMP-SMX and rifampin or streptomycin.
Discussion	Also called Malta fever, a microbial disease of animals, brucellosis is caused by several species of *Brucella*, a gram-negative, aerobic coccobacillus. It is transmitted to humans through the drinking of contaminated milk or through direct contact with products or tissues from animals such as goats, sheep, camels, cows, hogs, and dogs. The clinical picture is often vague; thus, a high index of suspicion may be necessary for diagnosis.

ID/CC	A 26-year-old female presents to the ER with intense, acute-onset left **lower quadrant crampy abdominal pain**, foul-smelling stools with streaks of blood, urgency, **tenesmus**, and fever.
HPI	For the past 2 days, the patient has also had headaches and myalgias. She frequently **drinks unpasteurized** ("raw") **milk** that she buys at a health-food store.
PE	VS: fever (39°C); tachycardia; normal RR and BP. PE: no dehydration; diffuse abdominal tenderness more marked in left lower quadrant.
Labs	Stool smear shows leukocytes (due to invasive tissue damage in the colon) and **gram-negative, curved bacilli**, often in pairs, in "gull-wing"-shaped pattern; dark-field exam shows motility; culture in microaerophilic, 42°C conditions on special agar yields *Campylobacter jejuni*, indicated by oxidase and catalase positivity.
Gross Pathology	Friable colonic mucosa.
Micro Pathology	Nonspecific inflammatory reaction consisting of neutrophils, lymphocytes and plasma cells with hyperemia, edema and damage to epithelium, glandular degeneration, ulcerations, and crypt abscesses caused by colonic tissue invasion of the organism.
Treatment	Self-limiting disease. Severe cases (i.e., high fever, severe diarrhea) can be treated with **fluoroquinolones**.
Discussion	One of the primary causes of "traveler's diarrhea." Sources of infection include **undercooked food** and contact with **infected animals** and their excreta. Prevent by improving public sanitation, pasteurizing milk, and proper cooking.

CAMPYLOBACTER ENTERITIS

ID/CC A 49-year-old morbidly **obese, diabetic** woman presents with **pruritus in the skin folds** beneath her breasts.

HPI She admits to having this problem chronically, especially in the warm summer months, when she perspires more heavily.

PE · Superficially **denuded, beefy-red areas** beneath breasts with satellite vesicopustules and **whitish curd-like concretions** on surface.

Labs Clusters of **budding cells with short hyphae** seen under high-power lens after skin scales have been put in 10% KOH; *Candida albicans* isolated in Sabouraud's medium.

Gross Pathology Rash has whitish-creamy pseudomembrane that covers an erythematous surface.

Micro Pathology Yeast invades superficial layers of epithelium.

Treatment Keep affected areas dry; clotrimazole or other antifungal agents locally.

Discussion Other superficial areas of infection include the oral mucosa (thrush), vaginal mucosa (vaginitis), and esophagus (GI candidiasis). Systemic invasive candidiasis may be seen with immunosuppression, in patients receiving **chronic broad-spectrum antibiotics**, in AIDS patients, or in those receiving hyperalimentation.

ID/CC A 25-year-old female presents with **painful lumps in her right axilla** and neck together with **low-grade fever**.

HPI Three weeks ago she was **scratched** on her right forearm **by her pet cat**; an erythematous pustule initially developed at the site but resolved spontaneously within 10 days.

PE VS: fever. PE: **tender right axillary** and cervical **lymphadenopathy**.

Labs Lymph node biopsy diagnostic; serologic indirect immunofluorescent antibody test for *Bartonella henselae* is positive.

Micro Pathology Hematoxylin and eosin staining reveals **granulomatous pathology** with stellate necrosis and surrounding palisades of histiocytic cells; **Warthin–Starry silver stain** reveals **clumps of pleomorphic, strongly argyrophilic bacilli**.

Treatment Symptomatic; fluctuant node may need aspiration; azithromycin given to immunocompromised patients.

Discussion *Bartonella henselae* is the agent that causes cat-scratch disease. Lymphadenopathy can persist for months and can sometimes be mistaken for a malignancy. Individuals who are immunocompromised may present with seizures, coma, and meningitis.

ID/CC	An 8-year-old white female enters the emergency room complaining of headache, malaise, and bipalpebral **swelling of the right eye**.
HPI	She recently returned from a year-long stay in **Brazil**, where her father works as a logger in the Amazon **forest**. Over the past week she had a high fever, which was treated at home as malaria.
PE	VS: fever (39°C); tachycardia. PE: right eyelid swollen shut (ROMAÑA'S SIGN); markedly hyperemic conjunctiva; **ipsilateral retroauricular and cervical lymph nodes**; hepatosplenomegaly.
Labs	PBS: **trypanosomes on thick blood smear**. ECG: right bundle-branch block; ventricular extrasystoles.
Gross Pathology	Encapsulated, nodular area (CHAGOMA) or Romaña's sign may be seen at point of entry, commonly the face.
Micro Pathology	Intense neutrophilic infiltrate with abundant macrophages at site of entry; myocardial necrosis with mononuclear cell infiltration; pseudocysts in infected tissues contain parasites that multiply within cells; denervation of myenteric gut plexus.
Treatment	Nifurtimox for acute disease.
Discussion	Chagas' disease is a parasitic disease that is restricted to the Americas (endemic in South and Central America) and is produced by *Trypanosoma cruzi*, a thin, undulating flagellated protozoan; it is transmitted by contamination of a **reduviid bug** bite with injection of its feces. Also known as American trypanosomïasis. Long-standing cases show myocardial involvement with **dilated cardiomyopathy**, life-threatening conduction defects, and apical aneurysm formation and may also show **megaesophagus or megacolon**.
Atlas Link	UCV1 M-M1-071

ID/CC	A 35-year-old male complains of **cough** productive of mucopurulent sputum and **breathlessness**.
HPI	Before the onset of these symptoms, he had a sore throat with hoarseness. He has no history of hemoptysis, sharp chest pain, or high-grade fever.
PE	Crepitations heard over left lung base.
Labs	CBC: normal leukocyte count. Sputum exam revealed no **bacterial organism**; microimmunofluorescence detected species-specific antibodies directed against *Chlamydia* outer-membrane proteins; cultivation of *C. pneumoniae* demonstrated on HEp-2 and HL cell lines.
Imaging	CXR: left lower lobe subsegmental infiltrate with interstitial pattern.
Treatment	**Doxycycline** is the drug of choice; **erythromycin** and **fluoroquinolones** may also be used.
Discussion	The peak incidence of chlamydia pneumonia is in young adults. The mode of transmission would appear to be from person to person.

ID/CC An 8-year-old male who recently emigrated from India presents with **bilateral eye irritation** and **photophobia**.

HPI He reports **recurrent episodes** of similar eye irritation and redness **in the past**.

PE Conjunctival congestion; **multiple (> 5) follicles**, each at least 0.5 mm in diameter, seen **in upper tarsal conjunctiva**; inflammatory thickening of tarsal conjunctiva; new vessels (PANNUS) seen in cornea at superior limbus; **punctate keratitis**.

Labs Diagnosis confirmed by demonstration of characteristic cytoplasmic inclusion bodies (HALBERSTAEDTER-PROWAZEK BODIES) in Giemsa staining of conjunctival scrapings.

Micro Pathology *Chlamydia trachomatis* is typically seen in conjunctival scrapings in colony form in the epithelial cells as H-P inclusion bodies. Histologically there is lymphocytic infiltration involving the whole adenoid layer of parts of the conjunctiva; special aggregations of lymphocytes form **follicles** that tend to show necrosis and certain large multinucleated cells (LEBER'S CELLS).

Treatment Topical **tetracycline** with systemic **tetracycline/doxycycline/erythromycin/azithromycin**; prophylaxis of family contacts with topical tetracycline.

Discussion *Chlamydia trachomatis* causes a variety of ocular diseases, including **neonatal inclusion conjunctivitis, sporadic inclusion conjunctivitis in adults, and sporadic as well as endemic trachoma**; trachoma is endemic in North Africa, in the Middle East, and among the Native American population of the southwestern United States. In endemic areas, trachoma is transmitted from eye to hand to eye, especially among young children in regions where standards of cleanliness are poor. Sporadic trachoma infection in nonendemic areas as well as sporadic inclusion conjunctivitis in adults results from transmission of the agent from the genital tract to the eye. Trachoma is a **major cause of blindness** in endemic areas.

Atlas Link [UCV1] M-M1-073

CHLAMYDIA TRACHOMATIS

ID/CC A 30-year-old man has sudden severe, **profuse (several liters per day) watery diarrhea, protracted vomiting**, and **abdominal pain**.

HPI He has just returned from a trip to **rural India**.

PE **Severe dehydration**; low urine output; generalized mild abdominal tenderness with no signs of peritoneal irritation; stools have characteristic **"rice-water" appearance**; (gray, slightly cloudy fluid with flecks of mucus), with no blood.

Labs Stool culture reveals gram-negative rods with **"darting motility"**; **O1 antigen detected**; *Vibrio cholerae* isolated on culture media; serum chloride levels decreased; serum sodium levels increased.

Treatment **Vigorous rehydration** therapy with oral and/or IV fluids; **tetracycline**, ciprofloxacin, or doxycycline.

Discussion A heat-labile exotoxin produced by *Vibrio cholerae* that acts by permanently **stimulating G$_S$ protein via ADP ribosylation**, resulting in activation of **intracellular adenylate cyclase**, which in turn increases cAMP levels and produces **secretory diarrhea**.

ID/CC A newborn baby is referred to the pediatrician for further evaluation of an unusually **small head**, low birth weight, and an extensive **erythematous rash**.

HPI **Intrauterine growth retardation** was prenatally diagnosed on ultrasound. The child's **mother had a flulike** episode during the **first trimester** of her pregnancy.

PE Small for gestational age; generalized hypotonia with sluggish neonatal reflexes; extensive **"pinpoint" petechial skin rash** (MULBERRY MUFFIN RASH); **microcephaly; chorioretinitis**; mild **icterus; hepatosplenomegaly; sensorineural hearing loss** in right ear.

Labs CBC/PBS: mild thrombocytopenia; atypical lymphocytosis. Moderately elevated direct serum bilirubin and transaminases. UA: cells in urine found to have large **intranuclear inclusions** (OWL'S EYE INCLUSIONS); cytomegalovirus isolated on tissue culture.

Imaging XR/CT, head: **periventricular calcifications; microcephaly**.

Treatment Ganciclovir (only for immunocompromised patients).

Discussion A congenital herpesvirus infection involving the CNS with eye and ear damage, congenital cytomegalovirus is a common cause of mental retardation.

ID/CC	A 13-year-old white female visits her pediatrician complaining of **fever**, severe **dyspnea**, and a **dry cough**.
HPI	She was recently diagnosed with acute lymphocytic leukemia, for which she received a **bone marrow** transplant. She is currently on **immunosuppressive therapy**.
PE	VS: fever; **tachypnea**. PE: pallor; **crepitant rales** over both lung fields; mild cyanosis; no hepatosplenomegaly.
Labs	CBC/PBS: anemia; leukopenia. ABGs: **hypoxemia**. No organism in induced sputum stained with Gram, Giemsa, ZN, and methenamine silver.
Imaging	CXR: diffuse, bilateral interstitial infiltrates.
Gross Pathology	**Interstitial pneumonitis**; hepatitis.
Micro Pathology	Characteristic **intranuclear inclusions with surrounding halo** (OWL'S- OR BULL'S-EYE CELLS) on transbronchial lung biopsy.
Treatment	**Ganciclovir** (CMV is resistant to acyclovir).
Discussion	An enveloped, double-stranded DNA virus belonging to the herpesvirus group; the most common cause of pneumonia and death in **bone marrow transplant patients**. It is also common in **AIDS patients**.
Atlas Link	UCV1 M-M1-076

ID/CC A 30-year-old homosexual white male presents to his family physician with a **rapidly progressive diminution of vision**.

HPI He is known to be **HIV positive** and periodically comes in for checkups.

PE **Cotton-wool exudates, necrotizing retinitis, and perivascular hemorrhages** on funduscopic exam.

Treatment Ganciclovir; foscarnet (CMV is resistant to acyclovir).

Discussion CMV retinitis is an important **treatable cause of blindness** that occurs in 20% of AIDS patients; 50% to 60% of patients develop retinal detachment within 1 year. Toxoplasmosis and progressive multifocal leukoencephalopathy (PML) are other important causes of blindness in AIDS patients.

CMV RETINITIS

ID/CC	A 19-year-old migrant worker from the **southwestern United States** is brought to the family doctor complaining of **cough, pleuritic chest pain, fever**, and malaise.
HPI	He also complains of a backache and headache along with an **erythematous skin rash** (due to hypersensitivity reaction) in his lower limbs.
PE	VS: fever; tachypnea. PE: central trachea; coarse, crepitant rales over both lung bases; tender, **erythematous nodules over shins** (ERYTHEMA NODOSUM); periarticular swelling of knees and ankles.
Labs	**Positive skin test with coccidioidin; dimorphic fungi** (hyphae in soil; spherules in body tissue); *Coccidioides immitis* on silver stain and sputum culture; positive latex agglutination test. CBC/PBS: eosinophilia.
Imaging	CXR: nodular infiltrates and thin-walled cavities in both lower lungs.
Gross Pathology	**Caseating granulomas**; often subpleural and in lower lobes; necrosis and cavitation may also be present.
Micro Pathology	Silver-stained tissue sections show spherules filled with endospores.
Treatment	Amphotericin B or itraconazole.
Discussion	Endemic in the southwestern United States, coccidioidomycosis is produced by *C. immitis* and is transmitted by **inhalation of arthrospores**. Systemic dissemination is frequent in blacks as well as in immunosuppressed and pregnant patients. Meningitis or granulomatous lung disease may result, which may lead to death.

COCCIDIOIDOMYCOSIS

ID/CC A 28-year-old male who lives in the **northwestern United States** complains of a high-grade **fever with rigors**, generalized aches, myalgias, headache, and backache.

HPI Four days ago he returned from a hiking trip during which he was **bitten by a tick**; he took amoxicillin as prophylaxis against Lyme disease.

PE VS: fever.

Labs CBC: leukopenia; relative lymphocytosis. Viral antigen detected in RBCs by immunofluorescence; **Colorado tick virus cultured** in suckling mice by intracerebral inoculation of blood clot; indirect fluorescent Ab test positive.

Treatment Symptomatic.

Discussion Colorado tick fever virus is an 80-nm double-shelled **reovirus** that is covered with capsomeres; its icosahedral core contains **12 segments of dsRNA**. The disease is a zoonosis that is transmitted by a wood tick, *Dermacentor andersoni*. It occurs primarily in the Rocky Mountain region, primarily affecting hikers. Since no specific therapy exists, prevention is key (wear clothing that covers the body).

ID/CC	A **2-year-old** male is brought to the ER by his parents with **sore throat, inspiratory stridor**, and a barking cough of 1 day's duration.
HPI	The patient has no significant past medical history.
PE	VS: fever (38.6°C); tachypnea. PE: **respiratory distress**; nasopharyngeal discharge; diffuse rhonchi and wheezes; examination of extremities reveals some cyanosis.
Labs	Throat and nasal swabs isolate **parainfluenza virus**; serodiagnosis and hemagglutinin inhibition tests reveal type 1 (most common cause).
Imaging	CXR: air trapping. XR, neck: **subglottic narrowing**.
Gross Pathology	Inflammation and edema of larynx, trachea, and bronchi.
Treatment	Most cases respond to **supportive therapy** such as humidified air, removal of secretions, and bed rest. Severe cases may require humidified oxygen, racemic epinephrine, or high-dose corticosteroids.
Discussion	Differentiate croup from *Haemophilus influenzae* type B and influenza A virus. Modes of transmission include respiratory droplets and person-to-person contact; tends to peak in the fall and winter. Most cases of croup are due to parainfluenza virus type 1; type 3 is a prominent cause of bronchiolitis in babies.

ID/CC A 30-year-old man with **AIDS** presents with chronic, recurrent **profuse, nonbloody, watery diarrhea**.

HPI The diarrhea has recurred over the past 2 months with intermittent cramping, and previous treatments have not been effective.

PE VS: no fever. PS: moderate **dehydration**; thin; generalized lymphadenopathy.

Labs **Acid-fast** staining demonstrates oocysts of *Cryptosporidium* in fresh stool.

Gross Pathology Intestinal mucosa appears normal.

Micro Pathology Blunting of intestinal villi; mixed inflammatory cell infiltrates with eosinophils in lamina propria; organisms visible on brush borders.

Treatment No treatment found effective; supportive management with maintenance of fluids and nutrition.

Discussion *Cryptosporidium parvum* infection presents as acute diarrhea in malnourished children and as severe diarrhea in immunocompromised patients (part of HIV wasting syndrome); the disease is mild and self-limiting in immune-competent patients. The disease is acquired through the ingestion of oocysts (fecal-oral transmission) that may be killed by chlorination.

Atlas Link 〔UCVI〕 M-M1-081

CRYPTOSPORIDIOSIS

ID/CC	A **5-year-old** white male presents with malaise, anorexia, low-grade fever, sore throat of 3 days' duration, and dyspnea on exertion.
HPI	The child was raised abroad. His immunization status cannot be determined.
PE	VS: fever; tachycardia with occasional dropped beats. PE: **cervical lymphadenopathy** (BULL'S-NECK APPEARANCE); smooth, **whitish-gray, adherent membrane over tonsils and pharynx**; no hepatosplenomegaly; diminished intensity of S1.
Labs	**Metachromatic granules** in **bacilli arranged in "Chinese character" pattern** on Albert stain of throat culture; *Corynebacterium diphtheriae* confirmed by growth observed on **Löffler's blood agar**; erythema and necrosis following intradermal injection of *C. diphtheriae* toxin (POSITIVE SCHICK'S TEST); immunodiffusion studies (Elek's) confirm toxigenic strains of *C. diphtheriae*. ECG: ST-segment elevation; second-degree heart block.
Imaging	Echo: evidence of myocarditis.
Gross Pathology	Pharyngeal membranes not restricted to anatomic landmarks; pale and enlarged heart.
Micro Pathology	Polymorphonuclear exudate with bacteria; precipitated fibrin and cell debris forming a **pseudomembrane**; marked hyperemia, edema, and necrosis of upper respiratory tract mucosa; exotoxin-induced myofibrillar hyaline degeneration; lysis of myelin sheath.
Treatment	Begin treatment on presumptive diagnosis; specific antitoxin and penicillin or erythromycin; respiratory and cardiac support; confirm eradication by repeating throat culture.
Discussion	A bacterial infection of the throat, diphtheria is preventable by vaccine and is caused by toxigenic *Corynebacterium diphtheriae*, a club-shaped, gram-positive aerobic bacillus. Diphtheria toxin is produced by β-prophage-infected corynebacteria; it blocks EF-2 via ADP ribosylation and hence ribosomal function in protein synthesis. The toxin enters the bloodstream, causing **fever**, **myocarditis** (within the first 2 weeks), and **polyneuritis** (many weeks later).

Atlas Links   UCV1 M-M1-082   UCV2 MC-324

ID/CC	A 56-year-old male professor of veterinary medicine from **New Zealand** experiences sudden **high fever** with chills, **jaundice**, and **right upper quadrant pain** while attending a conference in the United States.
HPI	His past history is unremarkable. He has been healthy and has been physically active working in the field with sheep and breeding **dogs**.
PE	VS: fever; hypotension (BP 90/50). PE: **hepatomegaly**; jaundiced sclera; on palpation of epigastrium and right hypochondrium, abdomen is tender with no rebound tenderness.
Labs	CBC: leukocytosis with neutrophilia; slight eosinophilia. Strongly positive **immunoblot test for antibodies to echinococcal antigens**; elevated direct bilirubin and alkaline phosphatase.
Imaging	CT/US, abdomen: **multiple large septated liver cysts** impinging on bile ducts, producing biliary dilatation (due to obstruction).
Gross Pathology	Liver is most common site of invasion, but cysts may also form in lungs, kidney, bone, and brain; each cyst contains millions of scoleces and consists of two layers: an inner germinal layer and an outer laminated layer; usually surrounded by fibrotic reaction.
Micro Pathology	Giant cell reaction surrounding cyst with eosinophilic infiltration.
Treatment	Surgically remove cysts if possible; albendazole may be effective.
Discussion	Echinococcosis is a zoonosis produced by *Echinococcus granulosus*. It is acquired through the ingestion of food or drink contaminated with the feces of dogs or other carnivores that have eaten contaminated meat; humans are the intermediate host of parasitic larvae. Accidental spilling of cyst fluid, either spontaneously or during surgery, may result in secondary seeding or anaphylaxis and even death. Also known as **hydatid disease**.
Atlas Link	UCV1 M-M1-083

ID/CC A 28-year-old male who is a resident of the **southeastern United States** presents with a high **fever with chills, headache, and myalgias**.

HPI He remembers having been **bitten by a tick** a week before developing his symptoms; however, he reports no skin rash.

PE VS: fever. PE: no skin rash noted.

Labs CBC: leukopenia and mild thrombocytopenia. **Characteristic intraleukocytic inclusion bodies** and serologic response to *Ehrlichia* antigens demonstrated; *E. chaffeensis* cultured from blood and detected by PCR.

Treatment **Doxycycline**.

Discussion Ehrlichieae are gram-negative, obligately intracellular bacteria. The two types of *Ehrlichia* species that affect humans are *E. chaffeensis* (which attacks macrophages and monocytes) and an *E. equi*-like organism (which attacks granulocytes). Preventive measures include wearing clothing that covers the body and using insect repellants.

ID/CC   A 30-year-old male from **Texas** presents with **fever and a skin rash** that began about 2 weeks ago.

HPI   The onset was gradual, with prodromal symptoms of headache, malaise, backache, and chills. These symptoms were followed by shaking chills, fever, and a more severe headache accompanied by nausea and vomiting. A remittent pattern of fever accompanied by tachycardia continued for 10 to 12 days, with the **rash appearing around the fifth day of fever**. The patient **worked at a rat-infested food-storage depot** this summer.

PE   VS: fever. PE: discrete, irregular pink **maculopapular rash** seen in axillae and on trunk, thighs, and upper arms; face, palms, and soles only sparsely involved; mild splenomegaly noted.

Labs   The **Weil–Felix** agglutination reaction for *Proteus* strain **OX-19 was positive**; complement-fixing antibodies to the typhus group antigen were demonstrated; **endemic typhus** (due to *Rickettsia typhi*) **was confirmed serologically** by using specific washed rickettsial antigens in IFA tests.

Treatment   Antibiotic treatment with **doxycycline** (**chloramphenicol** is used as an alternative).

Discussion   Murine typhus is a natural infection of rats and mice by *Rickettsia typhi*; **spread of infection to humans by the rat flea** is incidental and occurs when feces from infected fleas are scratched into the lesion. Cases can occur year-round; however, most occur during the summer months, primarily in southern Texas and California.

ENDEMIC TYPHUS

ID/CC	A 28-year-old Guatemalan male is brought to the hospital complaining of **severe headache**, photophobia, and fever over the past 2 weeks.
HPI	As a political dissident, he spent 4 months in a **refugee camp** in southern Mexico before entering the United States.
PE	VS: fever (40°C). PE: papilledema and delirium; bilateral swelling of parotid glands 1 week later; toxic facies; maculopapular **rash** on trunk and extremities; **face, palms, and soles spared**; mild splenomegaly.
Labs	**Positive Weil-Felix reaction** to OX-19 strains of *Proteus*; rise in complement fixation titer for *Rickettsia prowazekii*; specific antibodies. UA: proteinuria; microscopic hematuria.
Gross Pathology	Myocarditis and pneumonia may be present; cerebral edema; maculopapular rash.
Micro Pathology	**Zenker's degeneration of striated muscle**; thrombosis and endothelial proliferation of capillaries with abundant rickettsiae and perivascular cuffing; accumulation of lymphocytes; microglia and macrophages **(typhus nodules)** in brain.
Treatment	**Doxycycline**; chloramphenicol.
Discussion	Epidemic typhus is a febrile illness caused by *Rickettsia prowazekii*, a gram-negative, nonmotile, obligate intracellular parasite; it is transmitted via **body lice** and is associated with **war, famine**, and **crowded living conditions**. The rash should be differentiated from Rocky Mountain spotted fever, which starts peripherally on the wrists and ankles and also includes the palms and soles.
Atlas Link	·UCV2 MC-169

ID/CC	A **4-year-old** male presents with **fever, hoarseness**, and respiratory distress because of partial **airway obstruction**.
HPI	The child is also **unable to speak clearly and has pain while swallowing** (ODYNOPHAGIA).
PE	VS: fever; tachypnea. PE: **patient is leaning forward with neck hyperextended and chin protruding; drooling**; marked suprasternal and infrasternal retraction of chest; **inspiratory stridor** on auscultation.
Labs	Culture of throat swab (no role in management of acute disease) reveals penicillinase-resistant *Haemophilus influenzae*; blood cultures also positive.
Imaging	XR, neck: marked edema of epiglottis and aryepiglottic folds ("THUMBS-UP" SIGN).
Gross Pathology	Epiglottis is cherry-red, swollen, and "angry-looking." Rapid cellulitis of epiglottis and surrounding tissue leads to progressive blockage of airway.
Treatment	Preservation of airway; IV cefuroxime.
Discussion	The principal cause of acute epiglottitis in children and adults is *H. influenzae* type b; other pathogens include *H. parainfluenzae* and group A streptococcus. Characterized by rapid onset.
Atlas Link	UCV1 PG-M1-087

ID/CC	A 30-year-old soldier who had been admitted for a **gunshot wound** in the right thigh presents with **severe pain and swelling** at the site of his injury.
HPI	The patient's right lower limb had become discolored, and several bullae had appeared on the skin. He has passed very little urine over the past day, and the urine he has passed has been dark ("cola-colored").
PE	VS: low-grade fever; marked tachycardia. PE: diaphoresis; skin of right thigh discolored (bronze to purple red); site of injury exquisitely tender and tense and **oozing** a thin, dark, and **foul-smelling fluid; crepitus** while palpating thigh.
Labs	CBC: low hematocrit. Gram stain of exudate and necrotic material at wound site reveals presence of **large gram-positive rods**; anaerobic culture of exudate and blood yields *Clostridium perfringens* type A; culture isolate demonstrates **positive Nagler reaction** (due to presence of alpha toxin lecithinase); further labs confirm presence of **intravascular hemolysis, myo- and hemoglobinuria**, and **acute tubular necrosis**.
Imaging	XR, right thigh: presence of **gas in soft tissues**.
Gross Pathology	Overlying skin purple-bronze, markedly edematous with vesiculobullous changes with little suppurative reaction.
Micro Pathology	**Coagulative necrosis**, edema, **gas formation**, and many large **gram-positive bacilli** found in affected muscle tissue; relatively sparse infiltration of PMNs noted in the bordering muscle tissue.
Treatment	Surgical debridement; antibiotics (penicillin, clindamycin, tetracycline, metronidazole); hyperbaric oxygen therapy and polyvalent antitoxin; supportive management of associated multiorgan failure.
Discussion	A rapidly progressive myonecrosis caused by *Clostridium perfringens* type A, traumatic gas gangrene develops in a wound with low oxygen tension (embedded foreign bodies containing calcium or silicates cause lowering of oxygen tension, leading to germination of the spores). The most important toxin is the alpha toxin lecithinase, which produces hemolysis and myonecrosis.
Atlas Link	U C V 1 PG-M1-088

ID/CC A 4-year-old female is brought to the pediatrician because of **lack of appetite**; nausea and **vomiting; chronic, foul-smelling diarrhea** without blood or mucus; and a **bloated** sensation.

HPI She has been in several **day-care centers** over the past 3 years.

PE **Low weight and height** for age; mild epigastric tenderness.

Labs **Binucleate, pear-shaped, flagellated trophozoites** (*GIARDIA LAMBLIA*) on freshly passed stool; cysts found on stool exam.

Treatment Metronidazole.

Discussion The most **common protozoal infection in children in the United States**, giardiasis is transmitted mainly through **contaminated food or water** and causes malabsorption.

Atlas Links UCV1 M-M1-089A, M-M1-089B

ID/CC A **3-day-old** female neonate presents with a **thick eye discharge**.

HPI The **mother** admits to having **multiple sexual partners** and complains of a **vaginal discharge**. She did not receive adequate antenatal care.

PE Exam of both eyes reveals a **thick purulent discharge** and marked **conjunctival congestion** and edema; conjunctival **chemosis** is so marked that cornea is seen at bottom of a crater-like pit; **corneal ulceration** noted.

Labs Conjunctival swabs on Gram staining reveal presence of **gram-negative diplococci** both intra- and extracellularly in addition to **many PMNs**; conjunctival swab and maternal cervical culture yield *Neisseria gonorrhoeae*.

Treatment **Aqueous penicillin G** or **ceftriaxone** for a total of 7 days. Also treat mother and her sexual contacts. Educate the mother regarding the importance of safe sex.

Discussion Caused by *Neisseria gonorrhoeae*, gonococcal ophthalmia neonatorum is **contracted** from a mother with gonorrhea **as the fetus passes down the birth canal**; infection does not occur in utero. **Corneal inflammation** is the major clinical sign that may produce complications such as corneal opacities, perforation, anterior synechiae, anterior staphyloma, and panophthalmitis. It is now common practice to **prevent** this disease by treating the **eyes of the newborn with an antibacterial** compound such as erythromycin ointment or 1% silver nitrate; however, home childbirth bypasses this prophylactic procedure, and thus some cases are still occurring in the United States.

ID/CC	A 19-year-old white male presents with **burning urination**; profuse, **greenish-yellow, purulent urethral discharge**; staining of his underwear; and urethral pain.
HPI	Four days ago, he had **unprotected sexual contact** with a prostitute.
PE	**Mucopurulent** and slightly blood-tinged urethral discharge; normal testes and epididymis; no urinary retention.
Labs	Smear of urethral discharge reveals **intracellular gram-negative diplococci** in WBCs; gonococcal infection confirmed by inoculation into **Thayer-Martin medium**.
Gross Pathology	Abundant, purulent urethral exudate.
Treatment	Ceftriaxone plus doxycycline or erythromycin for **possible coinfection with *Chlamydia*.**
Discussion	A common STD caused by *Neisseria gonorrhoeae*, gonorrhea may involve the throat, anus, rectum, epididymis, cervix, fallopian tubes, prostate, and joints; conjunctivitis is also found in neonates. Neonatal conjunctivitis may be prevented through the instillation of silver nitrate or erythromycin eye drops at birth.
Atlas Links	UCV1 M-M1-091 UCV2 IM2-018

ID/CC   A 28-year-old male **immigrant** presents with **inguinal swelling** and a **painless penile ulcer**.

HPI   He admits to unprotected intercourse with **multiple sexual partners**, many of whom were prostitutes. He first noticed a papule on his penis several weeks ago.

PE   Soft, **painless**, raised, **raw, beef-colored**, smooth **granulating ulcer** noted on distal penis; multiple **subcutaneous swellings** (PSEUDOBUBOES) noted in inguinal region, some of which have ulcerated.

Labs   Giemsa-stained smear from penile and inguinal regions demonstrate characteristic **"closed safety pin"** appearance of encapsulated organisms **within a large histiocyte** (DONOVAN BODIES).

Micro Pathology   Characteristic histologic picture of donovanosis comprises some degree of epithelial hyperplasia at margins of lesions; dense plasma cell infiltrate scatters histiocyte-containing Donovan bodies.

Treatment   Treat with **doxycycline** or **double-strength TMP-SMX**.

Discussion   Granuloma inguinale, a slowly progressive, ulcerative, granulomatous STD involving the genitalia, is caused by the gram-negative bacillus *Calymmatobacterium granulomatis* (formerly *Donovania granulomatis*); it is seen in Giemsa-stained sections as a dark-staining, encapsulated, intracellular rod-shaped inclusion in macrophages, the so-called **Donovan body**. The disease is endemic in tropical areas such as New Guinea, southern India, and southern Africa.

ID/CC   A **60-year-old male** presents with **cough productive of mucopurulent sputum** together with mild fever and worsening breathlessness.

HPI   He is a chronic smoker who has been diagnosed with **COPD**.

PE   VS: fever. PE: in moderate respiratory distress; emphysematous chest with obliterated cardiac and liver dullness; **wheezing and crackles** heard over both lung fields.

Labs   *Haemophilus influenzae* organisms seen as small, pleomorphic gram-negative bacilli on Gram stain of sputum; **nontypable *H. influenzae* isolated on sputum culture** (to grow in culture, *H. influenzae* requires both factor X–hematin and factor V–nicotinamide nucleoside present in erythrocytes).

Treatment   **Amoxicillin/ampicillin therapy**; TMP-SMX, azithromycin, and clarithromycin are also excellent drugs for the treatment of clinically mild to moderate *H. influenzae* infections of the upper respiratory tract.

Discussion   Infections caused by nontypable, or unencapsulated, *Haemophilus influenzae* strains have been increasingly recognized in pediatric and adult populations. Nontypable *H. influenzae* strains are frequent respiratory tract colonizers in patients with COPD and commonly exacerbate chronic bronchitis in these patients; nontypable strains are also the most common cause of acute otitis media in children.

H. INFLUENZAE **IN A COPD PATIENT**

ID/CC A 25-year-old male presented with sudden-onset **breathlessness, cough, cyanosis, and high-grade fever**.

HPI The patient failed to improve on 100% oxygen, became hypotensive, and **died of type 2 respiratory failure** a few hours after admission. He had been in perfect health and had been **hiking in several rodent-infested areas** before falling ill.

PE On admission he was found to have fever, tachycardia, **cyanosis**, hypotension, and **rales on auscultation** over both lung fields; no meningeal signs or localizing CNS signs could be demonstrated.

Labs ABGs: respiratory acidosis with **hypoxia and hypercapnia**. CBC: leukocytosis; **hemoconcentration; thrombocytopenia**; atypical lymphocytosis. Increased LDH and ALT levels; prolonged PT index; sputum exam and blood culture did not yield any organism; IgM antibody to hantavirus and immunohistochemical stains for **hantavirus antigen in tissues confirmed** infection with the virus.

Imaging CXR: **noncardiogenic pulmonary edema** (bat-wing edema pattern).

Micro Pathology Histopathologic exam of lung tissues was suggestive of **acute respiratory distress syndrome** (adult hyaline membrane disease).

Treatment Patient died despite **intensive ventilatory support** (Sin Nombre virus most frequently causes hantavirus pulmonary syndrome in the United States).

Discussion A virus closely related to the **Hantaan virus** (which produces Korean hemorrhagic fever and hemorrhagic fever with renal syndrome) has been recovered from mice in various regions of the United States; **rodents are the natural host** for this group of viruses. Infected rodents shed the virus in saliva, urine, and feces for many weeks, and **humans** are believed to **acquire the infection via exposure to rodent excrement or saliva**, either by the aerosol route or by direct inoculation.

HANTAVIRUS PULMONARY SYNDROME

ID/CC   A 35-year-old male who works as a U.N. health worker presents with a high-grade **fever** and massive **hematemesis**.

HPI   He recently returned from **Zaire**, where he worked in a **tick-infested forest**.

PE   VS: fever. PE: extensive ecchymosis.

Labs   CBC: leukopenia; **severe thrombocytopenia**. LFTs: elevated AST. **Crimean-Congo virus isolated**.

Treatment   Treatment involves a 10-day course of **ribavirin; platelet transfusions; avoid salicylates**; barrier nursing and containment of infected secretions, since airborne infection may occur in hospital environment.

Discussion   The agent responsible for Crimean-Congo hemorrhagic fever is a **bunyavirus; reservoirs** include wild and domesticated **sheep, cattle, goats, and hares**. The disease is transmitted by a **tick vector, usually an ixodid** of the genus *Hyalomma*; endemic areas include the Middle East and western China. The disease targets individuals of all ages and affects males and females equally.

ID/CC   A 10-year-old male is brought to the ER in a state of **shock** accompanied by **massive hematemesis**.

HPI   The family had just returned from a vacation in **Thailand**. His parents say that he had a high-grade fever for 5 to 6 days, for which he was receiving presumptive treatment for malaria.

PE   VS: hypotension; tachycardia. VS: cool, clammy extremities; **petechial skin rash** over extremities, axillae, trunk, and face; bleeding from venipuncture sites.

Labs   CBC: **thrombocytopenia; hematocrit increased** by $> 20\%$. Abnormal clotting profile suggestive of **disseminated intravascular coagulation (DIC)**; paired sera reveal significant rise in titer of hemagglutination inhibition antibodies against **Dengue virus serotypes 1 and 2**.

Imaging   US: bilateral pleural effusion and ascites.

Treatment   Symptomatic; manage shock with fluids and hemodynamic monitoring; fresh blood/platelet-rich plasma; avoid salicylates.

Discussion   Dengue hemorrhagic fever is caused by a **mosquito-borne** (*Aedes aegypti*) **flavivirus** and is characterized by four distinct dengue serotypes (type 2 is considered the most dangerous). *A. aegypti* has a domestic habitat (stagnant water in flower pots, old jars, tin cans, and old tires) and bites during the day. Dengue fever has shown an increase in incidence in **Southeast Asia, Central and South America**, and the **Caribbean**. Since no specific therapy exists, prevent by avoiding contact with infected *A. aegypti*.

Atlas Link   UCV2 Z-M1-096

HEMORRHAGIC FEVER—DENGUE

ID/CC   A 58-year-old man who was hitchhiking through **central and southern Africa** was admitted to a hospital in Zaire in a state of shock following **massive hemorrhage from the GI tract** (hematemesis and melena); he died within 6 hours of admission. Ten days later, a male **doctor who had attended** this patient and had attempted resuscitation became **ill with a similar disease** syndrome.

HPI   At admission, he gave an 8-day history of progressive **fever, severe headaches, myalgias, and watery diarrhea**. He also reported an erythematous, **measles-like skin rash** that had begun to desquamate.

PE   VS: fever. PE: splenomegaly; hepatomegaly.

Labs   CBC: leukopenia; Pelger-Huët anomaly of neutrophils with atypical mononuclear cells; **thrombocytopenia with abnormal platelet aggregation**. Markedly elevated AST and ALT; blood was inoculated intraperitoneally into young guinea pigs and into various tissue culture cell lines, and **Ebola virus was detected by indirect immunofluorescent staining** techniques.

Gross Pathology   At autopsy, **lymph nodes, liver, and spleen** found to be most conspicuously involved (replication of Ebola virus can occur in virtually all organs); stomach and intestines filled with blood; petechiae seen over bowel mucosa.

Micro Pathology   Severe congestion and stasis of spleen; **widespread necrosis of liver** cells; **electron microscopy** of liver revealed **pleomorphic virus particles** appearing in contrast preparations as **long, filamentous forms, U-shaped forms, and some circular forms resembling a doughnut**.

Treatment   Supportive care, since no specific treatment exists; a prior outbreak was brought under control by isolating patients and instituting strict barrier nursing.

Discussion   A hemorrhagic, febrile infection of humans due to infection with the Ebola and Marburg viruses, both of which are filoviruses that are structurally indistinguishable but antigenically distinct. This disease is a zoonosis but the reservoir is unknown. Individuals can become infected through person-to-person or nosocomial contact.

ID/CC	A 25-year-old male woodcutter who lives in **South Korea** is admitted to the ER in a state of **shock and massive epistaxis**.
HPI	The patient had been complaining of fever, malaise, headache, myalgias, back pain, abdominal pain, nausea, and vomiting for the past week; he also complained of **extremely reduced urine output**. Careful history revealed that before he fell ill, he and his friend were cutting wood in the forest when they accidentally **disturbed a rodent-infested area**.
PE	VS: hypotension. PE: **epistaxis**; facial flushing; petechiae and subconjunctival hemorrhages.
Labs	Deranged RFTs suggestive of **acute renal failure**. CBC: **thrombocytopenia**. Serology and **culture identify hantavirus, Hantaan serotype**.
Treatment	Supportive management in the form of dialysis (**for renal failure**); management of shock and hemorrhage; **IV ribavirin** (must start within first 4 days of manifestation of disease).
Discussion	Korean hemorrhagic fever with renal syndrome is caused by **the Hantaan serotype of hantavirus**. Its reservoirs are various rodents that are found distributed over **Europe** and **Asia**; humans acquire the disease mainly by inhaling aerosols of rodent virus.

ID/CC	A **7-year-old** male complains of a **high fever** and a very **sore throat**.
HPI	The pain is so severe that the child refuses to swallow. He is adequately immunized and achieved normal developmental milestones.
PE	VS: fever. PE: **characteristic grayish-white vesicular lesions**, some of which have ulcerated, noted over **soft palate** and **tonsils**.
Labs	**Coxsackievirus A** isolated from mucosal lesions.
Treatment	Self-limiting condition.
Discussion	In **hand, foot, and mouth disease** (HFMD), patients complain of fever, weakness, and decreased appetite along with similar lesions noted in the oral cavity, palms, soles, and buttocks. Herpangina may be caused by coxsackievirus A1–A10, A16, A22, and B1–B5. Outbreaks of HFMD are usually caused by coxsackievirus A16.

ID/CC A 25-year-old homosexual male visits a health clinic complaining of headache, low-grade fever, and a **painful skin rash in the perianal area**.

HPI He has no history of penile ulcerations and admits to **unprotected anal sex** with **multiple partners**.

PE Perianal **vesicular** rash in clusters **on erythematous base**; no penile ulceration; painful inguinal lymphadenopathy.

Labs **Multinucleated giant cells with intranuclear inclusions** surrounded by clear halo on Pap-stained section or Tzanck preparation of scrapings from base of vesicles.

Gross Pathology Clear liquid in vesicles; secondary bacterial infection may result; painful ulcerations when vesicles rupture.

Micro Pathology Inflammatory infiltrate with abundant lymphocytes.

Treatment **Acyclovir.**

Discussion An enveloped, double-stranded DNA virus transmitted by sexual contact, HSV 2 has a **tendency to recur** and can be **transmitted to the fetus through the birth canal**. Condom use appears to be one of the most effective means of preventing transmission.

Atlas Links 🅄🅒🅥1 **M-M1-100**   🅄🅒🅥2 IM2-019A, IM2-019B

ID/CC	A 45-year-old **HIV-positive** male is seen by his family doctor following the appearance of a **painful, burning skin rash** on the **left side of his chest** that is accompanied by a headache and low-grade fever.
HPI	The patient had chickenpox as a child. He had been well until 1 year ago, when he was diagnosed with **non-Hodgkin's lymphoma,** for which he is currently undergoing **chemotherapy.**
PE	**Vesicular rash on erythematous base**; in **dermatomal distribution** (left T6–T8); exquisitely tender to touch.
Labs	Acantholytic cells on **Tzanck smear** from base of **vesicles.**
Micro Pathology	Intranuclear eosinophilic inclusions surrounded by clear halo (COWDRY A INCLUSIONS).
Treatment	Acyclovir.
Discussion	Shingles represents a reactivation of a latent infection with **varicella-zoster virus**; the rash typically follows the distribution of a nerve root. It is commonly seen in **immunosuppressed patients** and is also associated with trauma, ultraviolet radiation, hypothermia, and **emotional stress.** Postherpetic neuralgia is a common complication in the elderly.
Atlas Links	UCV2 IM2-020A, IM2-020B

HERPES ZOSTER (SHINGLES)